# Nursing Sk Cardiorespi Assessment and Monitoring

Organisms need to be able to maintain nearly constant internal environments in order to survive, grow and function effectively and efficiently. By maintaining homeostasis, humans remain healthy, strong and protected from the invasion of foreign organisms, such as viruses, bacteria and fungi. This practical pocket guide covers:

- the anatomy and physiology of cardiovascular system vital signs
- recognition of common arrhythmias and important skills for cardiovascular health cannulation and venepuncture
- the anatomy and physiology of the respiratory system
- skills related to addressing respiratory problems.

This competency-based text covers relevant key concepts, anatomy and physiology, lifespan matters, assessment and nursing skills. To support your learning, it also includes learning outcomes, concept map summaries, activities, questions and scenarios with sample answers and critical reflection thinking points.

Quick and easy to reference, this short, clinically-focused guide is ideal for use on placements or for revision. It is suitable for pre-registration nurses, students on the nursing associate programme and newly qualified nurses.

**Tina Moore** is a Senior Lecturer in Adult Nursing at Middlesex University, UK. She teaches nursing assessment, clinical skills and care interventions for both pre-qualifying and post-qualifying nurses. She is also a Middlesex University Teaching Fellow.

**Sheila Cunningham** is an Associate Professor in Adult Nursing at Middlesex University, UK. She has a breadth of experience teaching nurses both pre- and post-registration and she mentors clinicians supporting students in practice. She is also a Middlesex University Teaching Fellow and holds a Principal Fellowship at the Higher Education Academy. Her current role is Director for Learning, Teaching and Quality (School of Health and Education).

# Skills in Nursing Practice

### Series editors
Tina Moore, *Middlesex University, UK*
Sheila Cunningham, *Middlesex University, UK*

This series of competency-based pocket guides covers relevant key concepts, anatomy and physiology, lifespan matters, assessment and nursing skills for good clinical practice in a range of areas from safety and protection to promoting homeostasis. To support your learning, they include learning outcomes, concept map summaries, activities, questions and scenarios with sample answers and critical reflection thinking points.

Quick and easy to reference, these short, skills-focused texts are ideal for use on placements or for revision. They are ideal for pre-registration nurses, students on the nursing associate programme and newly qualified nurses feeling in need of a little revision.

### List of Titles:

**Nursing Skills in Professional and Practice Contexts**
*Tina Moore and Sheila Cunningham*

**Nursing Skills in Safety and Protection**
*Sheila Cunningham and Tina Moore*

**Nursing Skills in Nutrition, Hydration and Elimination**
*Sheila Cunningham and Tina Moore*

**Nursing Skills in Cardiorespiratory Assessment and Monitoring**
*Tina Moore and Sheila Cunningham*

**Nursing Skills in Supporting Mobility**
*Sheila Cunningham and Tina Moore*

**Nursing Skills in Control and Coordination**
*Tina Moore and Sheila Cunningham*

For more information about this series, please visit: www.routle dge.com/Skills-in-Nursing-Practice/book-series/SNP

# Nursing Skills in Cardiorespiratory Assessment and Monitoring

**Tina Moore and
Sheila Cunningham**

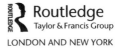

Routledge
Taylor & Francis Group

LONDON AND NEW YORK

First published 2021
by Routledge
2 Park Square, Milton Park, Abingdon, Oxon OX14 4RN

and by Routledge
605 Third Avenue, New York, NY 10158

Routledge is an imprint of the Taylor & Francis Group, an informa business

*British Library Cataloguing-in-Publication Data*
A catalogue record for this book is available from the British Library

*Library of Congress Cataloging-in-Publication Data*
Names: Moore, Tina, author. | Cunningham, Sheila, author.
Title: Nursing skills in cardiorespiratory assessment and monitoring / by Tina Moore and Sheila Cunningham.
Description: New York: Routledge, 2021. | Series: Skills in nursing practice | Includes bibliographical references and index. | Summary: "Organisms need to be able to maintain nearly constant internal environments in order to survive, grow and function effectively and efficiently. By maintaining homeostasis, humans remain healthy, strong, and protected from the invasion of foreign organisms, such as virus, bacteria and fungi. This practical pocket guide covers: The anatomy and physiology of the cardiovascular system Vital signs Recognition of common arrhythmias and important skills for cardiovascular health Cannulation and venepuncture The anatomy and physiology of the respiratory system Skills related to respiratory problems. This competency-based text covers relevant key concepts, anatomy and physiology, lifespan matters, assessment, and nursing skills. To support your learning, it also includes learning outcomes, concept map summaries, activities, questions and scenarios with sample answers, and critical reflection thinking points. Quick and easy to reference, this short, clinically-focused guide is ideal for use on placements or for revision. It is suitable for pre-registration nurses, students on the nursing associate programme and newly qualified nurses"–Provided by publisher.
Identifiers: LCCN 2020044614 (print) | LCCN 2020044615 (ebook) | ISBN 9781138479302 (hardback) | ISBN 9781138479326 (paperback) | ISBN 9781351066068 (ebook)
Subjects: LCSH: Respiratory organs–Diseases–Nursing. | Cardiopulmonary system–Diseases–Nursing.
Classification: LCC RC735.5 .M66 2021 (print) | LCC RC735.5 (ebook) | DDC 616.2/004231–dc23
LC record available at https://lccn.loc.gov/2020044614
LC ebook record available at https://lccn.loc.gov/2020044615

ISBN: 978-1-138-47930-2 (hbk)
ISBN: 978-1-138-47932-6 (pbk)
ISBN: 978-1-351-06606-8 (ebk)

Typeset in Stone Serif
By Deanta Global Publishing Services, Chennai, India

# Contents

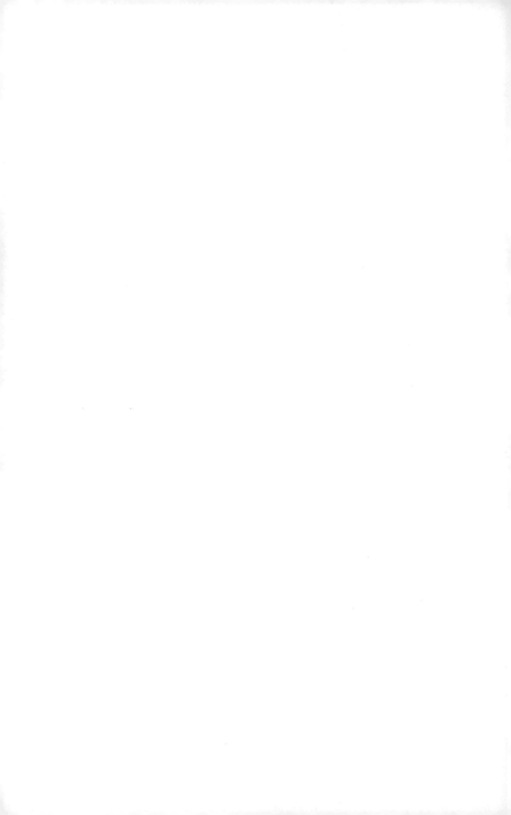

# Figures

# Introduction to the *Skills in Nursing Practice* series

This particular book is one in a series of six *'Nursing Skills in...'* books.

Book 1 *Professional Skills and Practice Context*
Book 2 *Protection and Safety*
Book 3 *Acquisition of Nutrients and Removal of Waste*
Book 4 *Control and Co-ordination*
Book 5 *Cardiorespiratory Assessment and Monitoring*
Book 6 *Supporting Mobility*

These books are designed to be used in clinical practice and can be used not only for reference but also as an invaluable revision tool. There is a continuing emphasis on skills acquisition and development particularly within nursing. This is accompanied by the increasing understanding of the necessity to effectively and efficiently integrate theory and clinical skill competence-based learning. In doing so, these books hope to ensure that nurses have the best opportunity to become fit to practice and develop key employability skills. Therefore, each chapter has been linked to the *Future Nurse Proficiencies* (NMC 2018) which will enable you to map your skills development in relation to the standards set by the professional body.

The structure of each chapter within the books draws on constructivist pedagogical approaches and assimilation theory. Each chapter presents interlinking ideas and information through the use of concept maps. It is anticipated that the use of key words and connections will deepen and enhance those linkages from the concepts, drawing on the general and specific aspects of a topic, and will therefore promote active learning.

1

Concept maps are pictures or graphic representations that will help you to organise and represent your knowledge of a subject. This is achieved through helping you to link, differentiate and relate concepts to one another. They (concept maps) begin with a main idea (or concept) and then branch out to show how that main idea can be broken down into specific topics. They can also visually represent relationships between concepts and ideas in a quick, easy-to-understand format. Concept mapping is becoming increasingly popular as a means of teaching and learning within education. The introduction of concept maps will provide a quick summary with additional key information about the material in the *Clinical Skills for Nursing* book. We have also included related anatomy and physiology together with lifespan matters.

The end of each chapter will have questions (answers also provided) in the format of a quiz. This will help you to test your new knowledge, understanding and application of the content. There is also the opportunity for you to critically reflect on your learning using the SMART (Specific, Measurable, Achievable, Realistic and Time-bound) format. From this you should then be able to clearly identify areas for future development and learning.

These pocket-size books are not only designed to help develop your clinical skills (practice and knowledge) but also to improve your key transferrable skills, enabling them to advance your employability skills, i.e. problem solving; analytical and critical thinking; and team working. Therefore another aim for each book is to concentrate on scaffolding learning, therefore supporting, promoting and developing autonomous learning, questioning (informed) and critical thinking. The use of concept mapping allows the reorganisation of information in a visual manner to promote critical thinking in the nursing student. Through concept mapping students can see how ideas and patient care needs, and the interrelationships that exist between them, promote critical thinking in relation to clinical practice.

The books within this series are not designed to be comprehensive textbooks. They are the practice companions of the *Clinical Skills for Nursing Practice*, and are designed to be used in conjunction with that book. The design of these 'pocket-size' books will enable students/readers to use them as a resource whilst working within and outside of clinical practice.

Tina Moore and Sheila Cunningham

# Introduction and overview

One of the traditional roles in nursing and arguably one of the most important is assessment and monitoring, which includes interpreting the assessment data and making quick and accurate intervention decisions. This might include monitoring patients for changes in their condition and recognising the early signs of clinical deterioration, in addition to the protection of the patient from harm or errors. The prompt detection and reporting of changes in vital signs are essential as delays in initiating appropriate treatment can detrimentally affect the patient's outcome and prognosis.

Today, in comparison to the past, there are increased survival rates: people are living longer but are becoming more sicker or are receiving more complex procedures and operations. In addition, their physiological illnesses are more complex and often pose more of a challenge to assessment, monitoring and care management for nurses and other health care professionals.

Assessment is the first stage in determining the patient's physiological health needs in the immediate, short and long term. It is the key to clinical decision-making and to planning patient care, taking into account the individual patient's needs and situation. The assessment process and careful monitoring of the patient's observations should facilitate early recognition of the patient 'at risk' (acutely/critically ill patient or one who is deteriorating / at risk of deterioration).

The data from the assessment should also aid in the correct identification of actual and potential problems, in addition to the prioritisation of care management. Approaches to assessment and the management of patients should be systematic, comprehensive and person-centred. In order to contextualise assessment, nurses must understand what the normal parameters are

3

for **that** individual patient. Remember too that, with chronic illness, there is a tendency for the patient to develop a level of physiological adaptation, so what is considered abnormal now becomes a 'new normal' for the patient.

It is also the responsibility of nurses and other health care professionals to carefully consider normal and baseline parameters together with acceptable targeted parameters for individual patients. This will enable them to interpret observations competently and make judgements about that data. This interpretation should lead to appropriate decisions and actions. All abnormal results should be escalated.

Vital sign observations should be recorded at the initial assessment and as part of routine monitoring (NICE, 2020). A clearly written monitoring plan should be available that provides information about which physiological observations should be taken and recorded and how often. A decision regarding the frequency of monitoring should be dictated by the patient's physiological condition along with a prediction of the patient's risk of deterioration; alterations in the frequency of observation should also be made by the multi-disciplinary team (MDT), taking into account if the patient is at the end of life and a Do Not Resuscitate (DNR) order is in place.

There are a number of frameworks (e.g. ABCDE, nursing models) available to help guide the assessment and process of care interventions. The ABCDE framework in particular is designed for those patients who become acutely/critically unwell or are at risk of physiological deterioration.

# CHAPTER 1

# Anatomy and physiology of cardiorespiratory system

*Sheila Cunningham*

## Overview

Cardiorespiratory systems are key to human functioning. For a body, optimal functioning depends on the individual and collective functioning of all cells. For optimal functioning, each cell depends on a stable supply of nutrients and oxygen and on the removal of waste. Working in unison to ensure such supply of essential items and removal of wastes is core to homeostasis and growth and development.

### Link to *Future Nurse Proficiencies* (NMC 2018)

*Platform 3* Assessing needs and planning care Section 3.2: demonstrate and apply knowledge of body systems and homeostasis, human anatomy and physiology, biology, genomics, pharmacology and social and behavioural sciences when undertaking full and accurate person-centred nursing assessments and developing appropriate care plans.

**Annexe B**: Nursing procedures Section 2: Procedures for assessing people's needs for person-centred care. Specifically 2.7: undertake a whole body systems assessment including respiratory, circulatory, neurological, musculoskeletal, cardiovascular and skin status.

## Expected knowledge

- The organs within the cardiovascular and respiratory systems
- Basic cellular needs and the concept of homeostasis
- The purpose of 'vital signs' and parameters within these for health.

## Introduction

Considerable information about the condition and functioning of the cardiovascular system can be obtained by examining a person's 'vital signs', which include pulse and blood pressure. The RCN (2017, 2) indicates that

> the monitoring and measurement of vital signs and clinical assessment are core essential skills for all health care practitioners working with infants, children and young people. This guidance applies to professionals who work in acute care settings, as well as those who work in GP surgeries, walk-in clinics, telephone advice and triage services, schools and other community settings.

Whilst this guidance focusses on children and young people it also vitally important for all clients in whatever situation and need.

At a cellular level, humans and cells have similar needs: oxygen and nutrients to carry out metabolic functions, and removal and excretion of wastes such as carbon dioxide and other waste products. The role of the cardiovascular system is to transport oxygen and nutrients to cells and remove waste, thereby maintaining a stable internal environment known as 'homeostasis'. In a complementary way, the role of the respiratory system is to take up oxygen and eliminate waste products from metabolism. As a unified team the cardiovascular and respiratory systems work dynamically together. Prior to performing associated skills, sound knowledge and understanding of these systems in terms of structure and function are essential.

## Content

| Cardiovascular functions | Control of blood pressure and heart rate | Regulation and homeostatic role of cardiovascular and respiratory systems |
|---|---|---|
| Respiratory functions | Control of breathing | Volumes and capacities |

## Learning outcomes

- Revisit the anatomical structures of the cardiorespiratory systems
- Differentiate lung volumes and capacities and why they are important in health monitoring
- Consolidate mechanisms and control of circulation and respiration
- Differentiate external and internal respiration and tissue needs including the role of microcirculation
- Reflect on knowledge of physiology and connections with nursing skills of monitoring vital signs.

## Key background

All life forms are comprised of connected units called 'cells'. This includes humans, animals and also some microorganisms such as bacteria. Like all living organisms, humans must maintain cell integrity and functioning to maintain life. Cells are not empty vessels but a complex blend of elements and components, namely chemicals, such as proteins, ions and other elements. This enables them to survive in very particular conditions and as such they are sensitive to changes in variables in the internal (as well as external) environment or 'stressors' such as changes in oxygen, heat or hydration. External and internal environments are constantly changing and impacting on cell and tissue functioning. Together with other stressors such as growth, ageing, diet and a wide variety of emotional and psychological triggers, environmental stressors can impact on physical functioning and disrupt performance. These can be translated into changes in processes or vital signs, or even to disordered functioning.

Normally, bodies are resilient in the maintenance of function (homeostasis) but when changes do occur they can manifest in a series of changes either physically (signs) or subjectively (symptoms) which can be observed or measured. As you may recall, stress is a key disruption to homeostasis and in the longer term can lead to problems such as behaviour changes (smoking, drinking, risky behaviours such as substance use) or ineffective coping mechanisms causing a 're-set' of normal functioning physiologically or even psychologically. Considering physiology, this may manifest as alterations in respiratory or cardiovascular functioning (i.e. heart rate, blood pressure, respiratory volumes or hyperventilation). Nurses can determine whether patients' health is improving or deteriorating by continually monitoring and evaluating their vital signs (Kim et al, 2017). These furnish objective measures of homeostasis and functioning. Vital signs are critical and nurses tend not to focus on them enough or give them enough priority.

One small study concluded that a nurse's ability to make clinical decisions is compromised by the lack of complete vital signs measurement, and pointed to the disastrous consequences of failing to detect deterioration in patients (Cardona-Morrell et al., 2016). A recent literature review (Brekke et al., 2019) raised the issue that among nurses and doctors there is insufficient knowledge and appreciation of changes in vital signs and their implications for patient care. The consequences of this are immense.

Prior to undertaking observations of vital signs and putting all the elements together to diagnose and help the individual, it is necessary to have a firm grounding in physiology. This will enable recognition not only of deviations from normal ranges of functioning but also of signs of deterioration in an acutely ill person or child. This chapter refreshes your understanding of cardiorespiratory physiology prior to a more detailed chapter on skills with vital signs and is an opportunity to consolidate knowledge to enhance nursing proficiency.

# CARDIOVASCULAR AND RESPIRATORY STRUCTURES

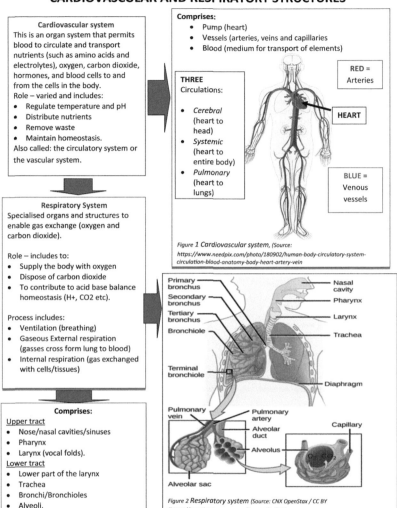

**Cardiovascular system**
This is an organ system that permits blood to circulate and transport nutrients (such as amino acids and electrolytes), oxygen, carbon dioxide, hormones, and blood cells to and from the cells in the body.
Role – varied and includes:
- Regulate temperature and pH
- Distribute nutrients
- Remove waste
- Maintain homeostasis.
Also called: the circulatory system or the vascular system.

**Comprises:**
- Pump (heart)
- Vessels (arteries, veins and capillaries
- Blood (medium for transport of elements)

**THREE** Circulations:

- *Cerebral* (heart to head)
- *Systemic* (heart to entire body)
- *Pulmonary* (heart to lungs)

RED = Arteries

HEART

BLUE = Venous vessels

Figure 1 *Cardiovascular system*, (Source: https://www.needpix.com/photo/180902/human-body-circulatory-system-circulation-blood-anatomy-body-heart-artery-vein

**Respiratory System**
Specialised organs and structures to enable gas exchange (oxygen and carbon dioxide).

Role – includes to:
- Supply the body with oxygen
- Dispose of carbon dioxide
- To contribute to acid base balance homeostasis (H+, CO2 etc).

Process includes:
- Ventilation (breathing)
- Gaseous External respiration (gasses cross form lung to blood)
- Internal respiration (gas exchanged with cells/tissues)

Primary bronchus
Secondary bronchus
Tertiary bronchus
Bronchiole
Terminal bronchiole

Nasal cavity
Pharynx
Larynx
Trachea
Diaphragm

**Comprises:**
Upper tract
- Nose/nasal cavities/sinuses
- Pharynx
- Larynx (vocal folds).
Lower tract
- Lower part of the larynx
- Trachea
- Bronchi/Bronchioles
- Alveoli.

Pulmonary vein
Pulmonary artery
Alveolar duct
Alveolus
Alveolar sac
Capillary

Figure 2 *Respiratory system* (Source: CNX OpenStax / CC BY (https://creativecommons.org/licenses/by/4.0)

**FIGURE 1.1** Cardiovascular and respiratory structures

# RESPIRATION AND BREATHING

**Ventilation and Perfusion**

**Ventilation** = the movement of air into and out of the lungs.
**Perfusion** = the flow of blood in the pulmonary capillaries.
**Gas exchange** = movement of gases across membrane – two sites (lungs and tissues).
- *External respiration* is the exchange of gases with the external environment (alveoli of the lungs).
- *Internal respiration* is the exchange of gases with the internal environment (tissues).
**Efficiency** - volumes in ventilation and perfusion should be compatible. Impeding factors: gravity effects on blood, blocked alveolar ducts, or disease can cause ventilation and perfusion imbalances.

**Gas Laws and Air Composition**

Gas molecules exert force on the surfaces with which they are in contact – *Pressure*.

The atmosphere – consists of oxygen, nitrogen, carbon dioxide, and other gaseous molecules: *atmospheric pressure*

**Partial pressure** ($P_x$) is the pressure of a single type of gas in a mixture of gases e.g. Oxygen has its own pressure.
Total pressure is the sum of all partial pressures. DALTON's LAW

Gas behaviour: gas moves from area of higher partial pressure to lower partial pressure.

**Atmosphere: sea level (example)**

All gases = 100% = **760mmHg**
Oxygen ($O_2$) = 20% = **159mmHg**
Nitrogen ($N_2$) = 78% = **597mmHg**
Carbon dioxide ($CO_2$) = 0.004% = **0.3mmHg**

**ALTITUDE**

Higher = lower pressure

Mount Everest = 260 mmHg
pO2 = 53 mmHg

Breathing deteriorates

**INSPIRATION/INHALATION**

Thoracic cavity expands.

External intercostals contract.

Diaphragm contracts

Figure 1 Breathing (Source: OpenStax College/CC BY (https://creativecommons.org/licenses/by/3.0)

**EXPIRATION/EXHALATION**

Thoracic cavity reduces.

External intercostals relax.

Diaphragm relaxes

INSPIRED pO$_2$ = 160mmHg

BLOOD: pO$_2$ = 104mmHg → TISSUE: pO$_2$ = 40mmHg   DIFFUSION

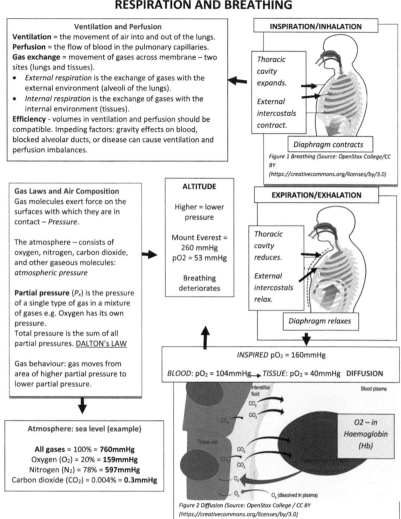

Figure 2 Diffusion (Source: OpenStax College / CC BY (https://creativecommons.org/licenses/by/3.0)

**FIGURE 1.2** Respiration and breathing

# RESPIRATORY VOLUMES AND CAPACITIES

Measures of movement of gas into and out of the lungs.

**Two types:**

1. Static (not effected by air flow):
**Volumes**
- tidal,
- inspiratory reserve,
- expiratory reserve,
- residual volumes.
**Capacities:**
- inspiratory,
- functional residual,
- vital capacity,
- total lung capacity.

2. Dynamic (air flow)
- mostly derived from vital capacity.
Dynamic lung volumes – obstructive lung diseases;
Static lung volumes – evaluation of obstructive or restrictive ventilatory defects.

**Tidal volume (Vt):** one cycle of inhalation/exhalation
**Inspiratory reserve (IRV):** the additional volume inhaled after tidal volume.
**Expiratory reserve (ERV):** the addition expired after tidal exhalation.
**Residual volume (RV):** the amount of air that remains in a person's lungs after fully exhaling.

**Inspiratory (IRC):** the maximum volume of air that can be inspired after reaching the end of a normal, quiet exhalation. The sum of the TIDAL VOLUME and the **INSPIRATORY** RESERVE VOLUME.
**Functional residual (FRV):** the amount of gas left in the lungs after normal exhalation.
**Vital capacity (VC):** the maximum amount of air a person can expel from the lungs after a maximum inhalation.

### FORCED EXPIRATORY VOLUME CALCULATIONS
**Forced expiratory volume (FEV)** measures how much air a person can exhale during a forced breath. The amount of air exhaled may be measured during the first (FEV1), or second (FEV2), of the forced breath. Can help in the diagnosis of a chronic lung disease, such as chronic obstructive pulmonary disease (COPD). When an FEV1 value is less than 80 percent of an FVC, it indicates an obstructive lung disease.

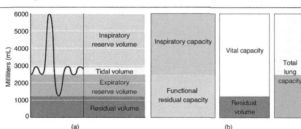

(a)          (b)
Figure 1 Volumes and Capacities (Source: OpenStax College/CC BY (https://creativecommons.org/licenses/by/3.0)

### PEAK FLOW
Also called: peak expiratory flow rate (PEFR)
- The amount and rate of air that can be forcefully breathed out after a full lung inhalation.
- Used to evaluate and monitor breathing problems (exhalation such as asthma).
- Emphysema or Chronic Bronchitis.

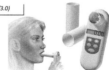

Figure 1 Spirometry (BruceBlaus/CC BY-SA (https://creativecommons.org/licenses/by-sa/4.0)

**FIGURE 1.3** Respiratory volumes and capacities

# RESPIRATORY REGULATION

### Control of Respiration
Breathing/respiration is required to sustain life.
- Involuntary respiration – not under direct, conscious control (brain stem).
- Involuntary respiration (Motor Cortex) allows it to happen when voluntary respiration is not possible, such as during sleep.

**Respiratory control centres** (brain):
- Medulla which sends signals to the muscles involved in breathing.
- Pons which controls the rate of breathing.

**Chemoreceptors:** in the medulla and in the aortic and carotid bodies of the blood vessels that detect changes in blood pH and signal the medulla to correct those changes.

### BREATHING Control = Balance of Inspiration and Expiration

### Medulla:
Two parts:
- *Ventral respiratory group –* **expiratory** movements.
- *Dorsal respiratory group –* **inspiratory** movements.
Also controls reflexes for non-respiratory air movements (coughing, sneezing, swallowing and vomiting).

### Pons:
Two areas:
- *Apneustic centre –* **inspiration** for long and deep breaths. It is inhibited by the stretch receptors of the pulmonary muscles and pnuemotaxic centre. It increases tidal volume.
- *Pnuemotaxic centre –* inhibit inspiration allows **expiration**. It decreases tidal volume.

- **Hyperventilation** causes **alkalosis**, which causes a feedback response of decreased ventilation (to increase carbon dioxide).
- **Hypoventilation** causes **acidosis**, which causes a feedback response of increased ventilation (to remove carbon dioxide).
- **Hypoxia** (too low oxygen levels) will cause a feedback response that increases ventilation to increase oxygen intake.
- Vomiting causes alkalosis and diarrhoea causes acidosis, which will cause respiratory feedback response.

### Consider this:
A young child has a tantrum and holds their breath to make you worry. What will happen?

**Answer:** the CO2 will build up and chemoreceptors will be stimulated which will cause the medulla to initiate involuntary inspiration. This overrides voluntary control.
This is not Acidosis but CO2 driven response to breathe (homeostasis).

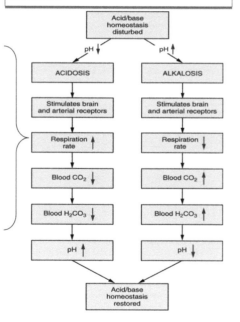

**FIGURE 1.4** Respiratory regulation

# CARDIAC CYCLE AND CIRCULATION

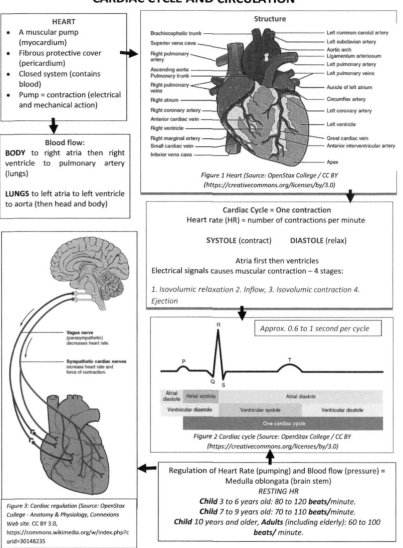

**HEART**
- A muscular pump (myocardium)
- Fibrous protective cover (pericardium)
- Closed system (contains blood)
- Pump = contraction (electrical and mechanical action)

**Blood flow:**
**BODY** to right atria then right ventricle to pulmonary artery (lungs)

**LUNGS** to left atria to left ventricle to aorta (then head and body)

**Structure**

Brachiocephalic trunk
Superior vena cava
Right pulmonary artery
Ascending aorta
Pulmonary trunk
Right pulmonary veins
Right atrium
Right coronary artery
Anterior cardiac vein
Right ventricle
Right marginal artery
Small cardiac vein
Inferior vena cava

Left common carotid artery
Left subclavian artery
Aortic arch
Ligamentum arteriosum
Left pulmonary artery
Left pulmonary veins
Auricle of left atrium
Circumflex artery
Left coronary artery
Left ventricle
Great cardiac vein
Anterior interventricular artery
Apex

*Figure 1 Heart (Source: OpenStax College / CC BY (https://creativecommons.org/licenses/by/3.0)*

Cardiac Cycle = One contraction
Heart rate (HR) = number of contractions per minute

SYSTOLE (contract)    DIASTOLE (relax)

Atria first then ventricles
Electrical signals causes muscular contraction – 4 stages:

*1. Isovolumic relaxation 2. Inflow, 3. Isovolumic contraction 4. Ejection*

**Vagus nerve** (parasympathetic) decreases heart rate.

**Sympathetic cardiac nerves** increase heart rate and force of contraction.

Approx. 0.6 to 1 second per cycle

R
P    T
Q
S

| Atrial diastole | Atrial systole | Atrial diastole |
| Ventricular diastole | Ventricular systole | Ventricular diastole |
| One cardiac cycle | | |

*Figure 2 Cardiac cycle (Source: OpenStax College / CC BY (https://creativecommons.org/licenses/by/3.0)*

*Figure 3: Cardiac regulation (Source: OpenStax College - Anatomy & Physiology, Connexions Web site. CC BY 3.0, https://commons.wikimedia.org/w/index.php?c urid=30148235*

Regulation of Heart Rate (pumping) and Blood flow (pressure) = Medulla oblongata (brain stem)
*RESTING HR*
**Child** 3 to 6 years old: 80 to 120 **beats/minute.**
**Child** 7 to 9 years old: 70 to 110 **beats/minute.**
**Child** 10 years and older, **Adults** (including elderly): 60 to 100 **beats/ minute.**

**FIGURE 1.5** Cardiac cycle and circulation

# CARDIOVASCULAR REGULATION

**Control of cardiovascular activity**

**Cardiovascular centre:** A region of the brain responsible for nervous control of cardiac output.
- *Cardioacceleratory centre* (CAC) – increases heart rate and stroke volume via sympathetic stimulation (cardiac accelerator nerve).
- *Cardioinhibitory centre* (CIC) – decreasing heart rate and stroke volume via parasympathetic stimulation (vagus nerve).
- *Vasomotor centre* (VC) – controls blood vessel tone, contraction and diameter. Effects peripheral resistance and blood pressure via sympathetic stimulation (epinephrine)

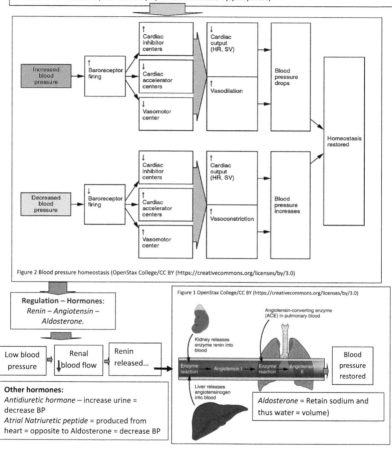

**FIGURE 1.6** Cardiovascular regulation

# BLOOD FLOW THROUGH THE BODY

## OVERVIEW

The primary purpose of the cardiovascular system is to circulate gases, nutrients, wastes, and other substances to and from the cells of the body. Movements across membranes vary:

- Small molecules (e.g. gases, lipids, and lipid-soluble molecules) diffuse directly.
- Glucose, amino acids, and ions use transporters to move through specific channels in cell membranes (*facilitated diffusion*).
- Larger molecules can pass through the pores of 'fenestrated capillaries', gaps or 'packaged' (*endocytosis and exocytosis*).
- Water moves by *osmosis*.

## What's the difference between tissue fluid and blood?

Blood consists of:

- Blood cells in plasma
- Dissolved substances including oxygen, carbon dioxide, salts, glucose, fatty acids, amino acids, hormones and plasma proteins.
- Cells include red blood cells(erythrocytes), white blood cell (leucocytes) and platelets.

Tissue fluid is:

- Similar to blood.
- Does not contain cells found in blood, nor does it contain plasma proteins.

## BULK FLOW

Mass movement of fluids into and out of capillary beds requires an efficient transport mechanism. *BULK FLOW:* comprising two pressure-driven mechanisms (**HYDROSTATIC PRESSURE** and **OSMOTIC PRESSURE**).

PUSH OUT and PULL IN

Hydrostatic pressure – blood in capillaries – capillary hydrostatic pressure (CHP) *PUSHES OUT* fluid from blood through capillaries to tissues
Tissue hydrostatic pressure - interstitial fluid hydrostatic pressure (IFHP) opposes CHP.
Process = **FILTRATION**

Osmotic pressure – osmotic gradient (concentration difference) principally plasma proteins – blood colloidal osmotic pressure (BCOP) and tissue osmotic pressure = interstitial fluid colloidal osmotic pressure (IFCOP). *PULLS IN* fluid.

## LYMPH...

- Not all tissue fluid returns to capillaries.
- Some is drained away into the **lymphatic system**.

## ROLE OF TISSUE FLUID

To transport and nutrients from the blood to the cells, and to carry carbon dioxide and other wastes back to the blood.

---

PUSH FLUID OUT

PULL FLUID IN

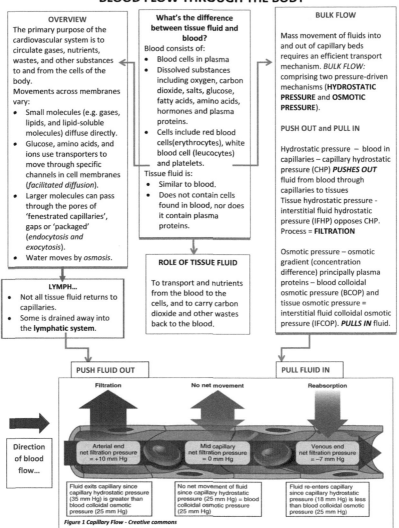

Figure 1 Capillary Flow - Creative commons

**FIGURE 1.7** Capillary exchange – microcirculation

## Activity: now test yourself

1. Blood which has been oxygenated by the pulmonary organs (i.e. which is leaving the lungs) is received back to the heart by the

    a) right ventricle

    b) left ventricle

    c) right atrium

    d) left atrium.

2. Oxygen and carbon dioxide are exchanged in the lungs and through all cell membranes. This is accomplished by which process?

    a) active transport

    b) diffusion

    c) osmosis

    d) filtration.

3. Which of the following regulatory chemicals involve or target the kidneys (tick all that are correct)?

    a) angiotensin

    b) aldosterone

    c) antidiuretic hormone

    d) atrial natriuretic peptide.

4. Referring to tissue fluid exchange, an increase in which **one** of the following results in increased filtration from capillaries to the interstitial (tissue) space?

   a) capillary hydrostatic pressure

   b) interstitial fluid hydrostatic pressure

   c) capillary osmotic pressure

   d) tissue hydrophobic force.

5. Atrial depolarisation (or systole) coincides in time with which of the following?

   a) P wave

   b) T wave

   c) QRS interval

   d) P-Q interval.

## Answers

1. c) right atrium.

   This is the receiving area of the heart and since this is the pulmonary circuit the route of blood is from the lungs to the heart. Recall that in the 'anatomical position', the directions 'left' and 'right' are the person's, not the observer's, left and right (i.e. as you look at the person head on, your right is the anatomical left).

2. b) diffusion.

   Active transport is against the concentration gradient, e.g. sodium–potassium pump.

   Diffusion is the process where molecules such as oxygen and carbon dioxide move from areas of high concentration to areas of low concentration.

   Osmosis involves the passive movement of water using the principle of diffusion but across a semi-permeable membrane.

   Filtration is when pressure is used to cross a membrane through which it separates suspended solid matter (cells/molecules) from a liquid. To do this the latter passes through the pores of some substance or permeable barrier called a filter. The liquid which has passed through the filter is called the 'filtrate', e.g. the kidney (glomerular) filtrate.

3. All are involved or target the kidney.

   Angiotensin is linked to the renin–angiotensin–aldosterone network and increases blood pressure by vasoconstriction.

   Aldosterone – as above, this hormone retains sodium and then water, thus increasing blood volume and blood pressure.

   The antidiuretic hormone inhibits water loss via the kidneys and increases blood volume and blood pressure, as above.

The *atrial natriuretic peptide* is released from the heart and the kidney, working opposite to aldosterone which increases the excretion of sodium and water, and thus reduces blood volume and ultimately blood pressure.

4.  a) capillary hydrostatic pressure.

    *The blood pressure entering the capillary is the capillary hydrostatic pressure and is the 'pushing out' force. Any capillary osmotic pressure is a 'pulling in' force. There is no interstitial hydrostatic pressure of note here and the hydrophobic force is a red herring!*

5.  a) P wave.

    *This is the start of the atrial contraction.*

**Reflection: ask yourself**

1. What do I know now that I didn't know before?

2. What am I confused/unclear about?

3. What areas do I need to focus on?

4. My action plan for further learning (make objectives SMART – (Specific/Measurable/Achievable/Realistic/Time-bound):

# CHAPTER 2

# Vital signs

Tina Moore

## Overview

'Vital signs', as the name denotes, are considered to be vital for sustainable life (Royal College of Medicine, 2019).

### Link to *Future Nurse Proficiencies* (NMC 2018)

***Platform 3*** Assessing needs and planning care (Sections 3.1; 3.2; 3.5).

**Annexe B, Part 1**: Procedures for assessing people's needs for person-centred care. Specifically, 2.1: take, record and interpret vital signs manually and via technological devices and 2.13: identify and respond to signs of deterioration and sepsis.

**Annexe B, Part 2**: Procedures for the planning, provision and management of person-centred nursing care. Specifically, 3.4: take appropriate action to ensure privacy and dignity at all times and 3.5: take appropriate action to reduce or minimise pain or discomfort.

### Expected knowledge

- Anatomy and physiology in relation to the cardiovascular system, respiratory system and temperature regulating centre
- Process of body heat production and heat loss
- Basic use of sphygmomanometer, stethoscope and thermometers
- Factors influencing assessment of the named vital signs
- Pulse points.

## Introduction

The four main measurements for vital signs are temperature, respiratory rate, pulse and blood pressure. Depending on point of view, pulse oximetry is considered to be (or not) the fifth vital sign. These vital signs in addition to assessing the level of consciousness are now part of the widely used National Early Warning Score (NEWS2) scoring system (RCP, 2017) and Paediatric Early Warning Score (PEWS). Work is currently being carried out by the Royal College of Paediatrics and Child Health (RCPCH) and the Royal College of Nursing (RCN) to produce a single national scoring system by the second half of 2021.

Measuring vital signs provides valuable information regarding the patient's physiological status, and in particular signs of deterioration. Following a repeat study, there is a noticeable improvement in the number of vital signs being recorded and monitored in the Emergency Department (ED) (Royal College of Medicine, 2019).

All patients have the potential to deteriorate physiologically, many of which cannot be predicted. It is important to note that not all patients will provide 'early warning signs' of that deterioration. In such cases, it is impossible for prediction to occur. For this reason, the taking, recording and in particular monitoring of physiological vital signs is essential.

## Content

| Related physiology | Procedure for taking temperature, pulse, blood pressure and respiratory assessment | Normal parameters |
|---|---|---|
| Factors influencing normal measurements | Significance of abnormal measurements | |

## Learning outcomes

- Demonstrate knowledge, understanding and skill in undertaking assessments of temperature, pulse, blood pressure and respiration

- Correct use of appropriate equipment including thermometer and sphygmomanometer
- Analyse data obtained from observations
- Identify and explain factors that influence the assessment of vital signs.

## Key background

The assessment of vital signs includes temperature, blood pressure, pulse (heart rate) and breathing rate, and has in many clinical settings been expanded to include oxygen saturation. Vital signs should act as baseline indicators of a patient's health status. Vital signs are in no way passive; there are many influencing factors to consider when interpreting vital signs such as pain, anxiety and circadian rhythms.

As part of a National Quality Improvement Project, the Royal College of Emergency Medicine (2019) reported that there were significant improvements in the repeat measurements of vital signs and subsequent action taken in comparison to the last audit results in 2010/2011. The Royal College of Emergency Medicine has produced standards for the taking, recording and monitoring of vital signs. Whilst predominately designed for the emergency departments, these standards can be transferred to any care setting.

Investigations are being made into technology that can assist nurses to reduce the workload and time spent taking vital signs, thus improving efficiency and effectiveness. At the timing of writing, NICE has produced a summary document outlining a digitalised approach to taking and recording vital signs.

This technology is designed not to make direct contact with people or medical hardware and uses algorithms to analyse the measurements. This may prove to be useful in limiting cross contamination. However, there are concerns with this approach, namely that other subtle assessment data such as the pulse volume or skin perfusion will not be assessed or readily available via a machine. There is a school of thought that believes that vital signs should be taken manually and not copied from a monitor. This development is still in the early stages of its advancement. At the time of writing, there is no published evidence to support or disprove its usefulness or evaluation.

The competent clinical assessment of vital signs in a timely manner together with early detection (using a proactive approach) should help to identify those patients who are at risk or who are physiologically deteriorating. This process is assisted by the use of scoring systems, namely the National Early Warning Scores / Paediatric Early Warning Score (NEWS2/PEWS).

Physiological changes are determined by the patient's vital signs, i.e. blood pressure; pulse (rate, rhythm and depth); respiration (rate, rhythm and depth); oxygen saturation levels; level of consciousness; and temperature. The scoring system identifies those who are at serious risk of clinical deterioration and poor clinical outcome and who need urgent further assessment and intervention. It is anticipated that the decision-making ability of the user (mainly nurses) would then be enhanced by enabling them to reach a conclusion of clinical deterioration. It is anticipated that this recognition should be quick and lead to a more timely and appropriate intervention. Such tools include National Early Warning Scores (NEWS2) (Royal College of Physicians, 2017) and the track and trigger scoring system (Royal College of Physicians, 2017). These observation tools have continued to gain momentum in their implementation (NICE, 2007; NPSA, 2007; Royal College of Physicians, 2017).

Nurses should ensure that they are competent in performing these skills. There are many influencing factors of which the outcomes could be a false high score or a false low score. The results are important and significant as treatment is often initiated/altered on these results. So, not only is knowledge and understanding important but so are psychomotor skills.

# TEMPERATURE (ORAL/AXILLARY)

Heat is produced as a by-product of cellular metabolism and is lost through the mechanisms of:

**Radiation** – transfer of heat without contact between the surfaces of both objects (e.g. infrared rays, like sun rays).

**Convection** – process of losing heat through the movement of air or water molecules across the skin (e.g. use of a fan).

**Conduction** – transfer of heat through physical contact with another object or body of a lower temperature (e.g. when touching, heat from one person would transfer to the colder person).

**Vaporisation** – evaporation of moisture from the skin, mouth and respiratory tract. Heat is lost through the conversion of water to gas (respiration).

Additional observations should also be performed e.g. skin temperature (cold, warm, hot or sweaty), shivering or huddled in a ball to try and keep warm. Children under three are vulnerable to seizures (febrile convulsion) resulting from a high temperature.

Normal body temperature is considered to be:

| | |
|---|---|
| Oral | 36.5°C–37.5°C (NICE, 2008) |
| Axilla | 36.0°C–36.7°C |
| Tympanic | 37.5°C |
| Rectal | 36.2°C–37.7°C |

**Procedure for taking an oral temperature**

Never use this route for patients who are confused, unpredictable, semi- or unconscious, recovering from facial/oral surgery, have damage to the mouth, teeth and face (including sores), dyspnoeic, under 5 years old.

1. Prior to this procedure, the patient should not have ingested any hot or cold fluids orally, or have been smoking for at least 30 minutes.
2. Wash and dry hands before and after procedure. Explain procedure. Where possible gain consent.
3. With the silver end of the thermometer pointing downwards, hold firmly at the clear end, use wrist movement to flick it quickly a few times. This will move the alcohol (silver line in the middle) to the bottom.
4. There is no need to shake the digital thermometers. The result is displayed on the liquid crystal display (LCD) screen. It is important to ensure that it is switched on and that the screen is clear from old readings.
5. Ask the patient to open their mouth and curl up their tongue.
6. Place the thermometer (the silver tip end) under the tongue (posterior sublingual pocket of tissue).
7. The patient should close their mouth around the thermometer (being careful not to bite it). Leave the thermometer in place as guided by the manufacturers (alcohol thermometer, a minimum of three minutes; single use, one minute minimum). The digital thermometers will give a 'beeping' sound when ready. Look at the thermometer: where the silver line has stopped (on the graduated line), that is the temperature.
8. Clean the thermometer with an antiseptic (follow manufacturer's guidance) and store in an appropriate container (usually plastic) to prevent breakage, or discard the covering sheath, this reduces the risk of infection.
9. Document findings.

**Procedure for taking an axillary temperature**

Do not perform this procedure on patients who are emaciated or who are obese. Note that this method provides the least accurate results.

1. Wash hands before and after the procedure.
2. Explain procedure and where possible gain consent.
3. Maintain patient's privacy and dignity.
4. Ask the patient to elevate their elbow to expose the axilla. If they cannot do this, *gently manually elevate this arm (taking care to support the elbow).*
5. Ensure the axilla is clean and dry.
6. The silver tip of the thermometer should be placed vertically under the right armpit.
7. Close the arm over the thermometer so that it is firmly against the chest, making it secure.
8. Follow manufacturer's guidance for how long the thermometer should stay in place (a minimum of seven minutes for alcohol thermometer; three minutes for single use). Document findings.
9. Remove and read the thermometer.

**FIGURE 2.1** Temperature (oral/axillary)

# TEMPERATURE (TYMPANIC/RECTAL)

**Procedure for taking a tympanic temperature (ear drum)**

Recommended for use with children under 5 years (NICE 2013).

Do not use on patients following aural (ear) surgery or those with excessive ear wax/ear discharge.

**The procedure.** This is a quick procedure.

1. Wash/dry hands before and after procedure.
2. Explain procedure and where possible gain consent.
3. Use play techniques with children to gain co-operation.
4. Place the disposable cover over the probe.
5. Instruct the patient to keep their head still, gently pull the earlobe up then back and insert the probe into the ear canal. DO NOT FORCE THE PROBE. After 1–2 seconds a beeping sound will indicate when the results are ready.
6. Remove the thermometer and discard the disposable cover.
7. Record findings.

**Procedure for taking a rectal temperature**

Closest to the core body temperature and therefore most accurate. This route should not be routinely performed on children (NICE, 2013) and never on babies of less than six months. Student nurses should always be supervised when taking a rectal temperature because of the risk of perforating the rectum. For the same reasons, this procedure should not be performed on patients who have irritation to their large bowel (e.g. bowel perforation), recently undergone rectal surgery, those who have diarrhoea or haemorrhoids and those with clotting disorders (can haemorrhage very easily). Do not take a rectal temperature on a patient who has a cardiac condition. The thermometer/probe could stimulate the vagus nerve in the rectum and cause cardiac arrhythmias.

**The procedure**

1. Wash/dry hands before and after procedure.
2. Explain procedure and where possible gain consent.
3. Maintain patient's privacy and dignity.
4. Patient should lie in the left lateral position if possible.
5. Expose the buttocks only (maintain privacy and dignity).
6. Ensure that the rectal area is clean and dry.
7. Use thermometers designed solely for the use of the rectum (some may have a sheath).
8. With a non-sterile gloved hand hold the thermometer and lubricate the first third.
9. Insert up to 1.5 cm of the thermometer very gently inside the rectum - DO NOT FORCE THE THERMOMETER IN PLACE.
10. The patient may contract their buttocks, try to reassure them/distract them if possible.
11. Hold the thermometer in place until the end of the procedure, which should take approximately three minutes (follow the manufacturer's guidance for length of time).
12. Wipe lubrication from the rectal area and thermometer.
13. Allow patient to get dressed.
14. Clean the thermometer with an antiseptic (follow manufacturers guidance) and store in an appropriate container. If the thermometer has a sheath – discard.
15. Document findings.

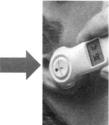

**FIGURE 2.2** Temperature (tympanic/rectal)

# PULSE

## Pulse assessment should consider:

**Rate** – involves the sympathetic and parasympathetic nerves; hormones (epinephrine or norepinephrine).

**Rhythm** – should be regular (some patients may have long term arrhythmias e.g. atrial fibrillation.) Any changes to 'normal' rhythm should be reported immediately. Note if the pulse has a regular, irregular or regular irregular pattern. Irregular patterns feel erratic, unsteady and uneven. Regular irregular patterns are regular patterns overall with 'skipped' (missed) beats.

**Volume** – if blood volume is low, pulse volume will be low (weak and thready). A slow pulse may indicate a high stroke volume, and as there is a long time between each ejection of blood, the pulse pressure (the difference between systolic and diastolic pressure) will be high.

|  | **Awake** | **Asleep** |  |
|---|---|---|---|
| <28 days | 100 - 205 | 90 – 160 | bpm |
| 1-12 mos | 100-190 | 90-160 | |
| 1-2 ys | 98-140 | 80-120 | |
| 3-5 ys | 80-120 | 65-100 | |
| 6-11 ys | 75-118 | 58-90 | |
| 12- Ault | 60-100 | 50-90 | |
| Athletes | 40 - 60 | | |

PALS (2015)

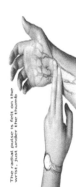

The radial pulse is felt on the wrist, just under the thumb

## Causes of Tachycardia

**Emotion** (anger/excitability) – sympathetic nerve stimulated. Accompanied by a surge of adrenaline into the circulation.

**Exercise** releases epinephrine and lactic acid.

**Drugs** – e.g. bronchodilators, thyroxine, anti-depressants, amphetamines.

**Temperature** – increases metabolic rate.

**Shock** – vasoconstriction caused by increased sympathetic nervous activity and release of adrenaline.

**Hypoxaemia** – increased sympathetic activity used to distribute oxygen.

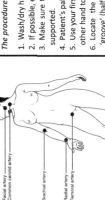

Temporal artery
Facial artery
Common carotid artery
Brachial artery
Radial artery
Femoral artery
Popliteal artery
Posterior tibial artery
Dorsalis pedis artery

Pulse points

## Causes of Bradycardia

**Cardiac dysrhythmias** – particularly problems associated with sinoatrial or atrialventricular nodes.

**Hypothermia** causes decreased impulses from the sinoatrial node.

**Disorders of the nervous system /neurological insult** – impairs control of autonomic nervous system (sympathetic and parasympathetic nerves).

**Drugs** e.g. beta-blockers (reduces the effects of epinephrine).

## The procedure

1. Wash/dry hands before and after procedure.
2. If possible, explain the procedure and obtain consent.
3. Make sure the limb (normally the forearm and hand) is supported.
4. Patient's palm should be turned upward.
5. Use your first two fingertips (index and middle) from your other hand to locate the pulse.
6. Locate the thumb and slide your fingers down the 'groove' (halfway between the tendons that run down the centre of your forearm and the edge of the patient's arm).
7. Ensure your fingers are vertical and not one finger on 'stacked' on top of each other.
8. Press firmly (not too hard). You will feel a pulsating motion under your fingers. Count the number of beats for a whole minute. Also noting the strength and rhythm of the pulse).
9. Document your findings.

**FIGURE 2.3** Pulse

**Procedure for taking a blood pressure (Preparation of patient)**

1. Ideally, the patient should rest for 5 minutes prior (this may be unsafe).
2. Note any influencing factors e.g., distress, pain or had eaten a meal, alcohol or smoked 30 minutes prior (may increase blood pressure), Children, sucking, crying and eating can also influence results and should be documented. If possible manage the influencing factor (e.g. analgesia).
3. Explain procedure and gain consent if possible.
4. If this is the first recording, if possible, take and record the blood pressure on both limbs. If there is a difference of more than 10mmHg this should be escalated.
5. The limb should be free from any clothing as this will provide false results. Maintain privacy and dignity.
6. The patient should not cross their legs (can increase blood pressure).

# BLOOD
# PRESSURE (B/P)

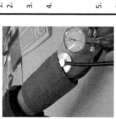

**Lying and standing B/P**

This is performed to assess postural hypotension. Due to the risk of dizziness and fainting, caution should be taken to maintain patient safety.

1. Wash/dry hands before and after procedure.
2. Explain procedure to the patient and where possible gain consent.
3. Record lying B/P first (patient should lie supine for approximately 10 minutes).
4. Allow sufficient time for the position change to standing (patient should stand for one minute (NICE, 2020)) before measuring the B/P. If the patient cannot stand, record the B/P in the sitting position (legs hanging down at the edge of the bed).
5. If the patient complains of feeling dizzy – put them in the supine position. Immediately then take the B/P.
6. Escalate and document findings.

**The Procedure** (Manufacturer's guidance should be followed when using any device) – Patient should be in an upright position if possible.

1. Ensure that the device is working properly with no faults.
2. Cuff size should be: the circumference of the patient's limb (normally upper arm) is used to determine this. The cuff width should be 40% of the limb circumference, and the length should be 80% of the circumference of the patient's limb.
3. Cuff sizes are infant, child/paediatric, small adult, adult, and large adult (i.e. 45cm). If the cuff is too small, it will over inflate, over constrict and be very uncomfortable (result = false high). If the cuff is too large it will move around the arm (result = false low).
4. Wash/dry hands before and after the procedure. Ideally, use the same arm each time. Avoid using the arm with intravenous fluids administered or pulse oximetry readings.
5. Feel the patient's pulse. If the pulse is irregular, use a manual device NOT an automated device (NICE, 2019) as recordings may be inaccurate.
6. For manual recordings, the arm should be slightly flexed and with the palm of the hand facing upwards and supported (table if possible). The position should be at the same level as the heart. An arm below the level of the heart causes a decrease in B/P. If the arm is above the level of the heart it causes an increase in B/P.
7. Completely deflate and squeeze the air out of the cuff ensuring it is free from any trapped air.
8. Apply the cuff (arrow) over the brachial artery. The cuff should be approximately 2.5 cm above the antecubital fossa
9. Place the device at the same level as the limb.
10. Identify the systolic pressure. Close the valve and with the other hand, palpate the radial pulse. Inflate the cuff until the pulse disappears. Note the reading on the dial. Deflate the cuff quickly and fully.
11. Locate the brachial pulse and inflate the cuff to 20–30 mmHg above the predicted systolic reading, release the pressure slowly and controlled (deflation rate of 2–3mmHg per second (NICE, 2011)). The sound phases you need to identify are the first (systolic) and last (diastolic) sounds (Korotkoff).
12. Once the very last sound is heard, continue to deflate quickly ensuring all air has been removed from the cuff and record findings.
13. Follow local policy to clean the equipment.
14. It is necessary to recheck the B/P if there are significant differences from the last reading. Report any significant changes.

**FIGURE 2.4** Monitoring blood pressure

# BLOOD PRESSURE 2

B/P is dependent upon cardiac output (CO) and systemic vascular resistance (SVR). Therefore, B/P = CO X SVR

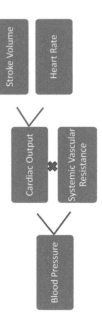

Stroke Volume

Heart Rate

Cardiac Output

Systemic Vascular Resistance

Blood Pressure

**Factors affecting blood pressure** (physiological, social, psychological origins).

Note: **A child's blood pressure** varies with age and is closely related to height and weight. Emotional states including pain, may result in a rise in actual B/P.

For the adult factors can also include:

**Contraction** – a weak myocardium can cause a reduced stroke volume, cardiac output and hypotension.

**Systemic Vascular Resistance** – vasoconstriction (e.g. shock) can result in an temporary increase in B/P. Vasodilatation can cause hypotension (reduced pre load).

**Disease process** – e.g. arteriosclerosis (hypertension).

**Blood volume** – a reduction causes hypovolaemia. Equally, an increase (fluid retention) can cause hypertension.

**Anxiety/stress/emotions/pain** – influence of catecholamine causing tachycardia and hypotension.

**Diet** – too much salt (causes fluid retention), alcohol and caffeine increases blood pressure.

**Ethnicity** – Afro-Caribbean and Asian origins have higher incidence of hypertension.

**Drugs** – many medications can either increase or decrease blood pressure (e.g. Ibuprofen can increase/ diuretics can decrease).

**Gender** – women who are premenopausal have a lower blood pressure than men of the same age. Those who are postmenopausal have a higher blood pressure.

**Age** – blood pressure gradually increases with age (atherosclerotic changes).

**Diurnal variations** – blood pressure peaks in the late afternoon/evening and is at its lowest in the early hours of the morning (during deep sleep).

## Normal blood pressure

B/P increases throughout the aging process. Within the literature there are inconsistencies as to what constitutes a 'normal' range of blood pressure for children.

| | Systolic (mmHg) | Diastolic (mmHg) |
|---|---|---|
| 1–12 months | 72–104 | 37–56 |
| 1–2 years | 86–106 | 42–63 |
| 3–5 years | 89–112 | 46–72 |
| 6 – 9 years | 97–115 | 57–76 |
| 10–11 years | 102–120 | 61–80 |
| 12–15 years (PALS, 2015) | 110–131 | 64–83 |
| Adult | 140 | 90 |

**Factors affecting blood pressure recording:**

*Poor technique* – Incorrect procedure; failing to follow recommend guidance by the manufacturer; incorrect size of cuff; leaks, kinks and twists present in the stethoscope.

*Faulty equipment* – Poorly maintained and calibrated equipment. Worn/torn bladder and cuff. Leaks in the outlet valve or tubing.

**FIGURE 2.5** Blood pressure 2

# RESPIRATORY ASSESSMENT

Ensure a well illuminated environment that is not too cold. Minimal distraction to nurse and patient. If able, the patient should be in an upright position (remember to document position). Consent may be required e.g. accessing patient's bare chest.

| Age | Rate |
|---|---|
| New born–1 year | 30–60 |
| 1–3 years | 24–40 |
| 4–5 years | 22–34 |
| 6–12 years | 18–30 |
| Adolescent | 12–16 |
| (Fleming et al, 2011) | |
| Adult | 12–20 |

What is considered to be normal parameters within the literature is variable.

**Rate:** If required and able, allow patient to rest for 5 minutes before counting. Observe movement of the chest, one breath = inhalation-exhalation. Count for 1 full minute (particularly for the child), allowing for any irregular breathing patterns.

**Tachypnoea** – higher than the normal rate. This is the most common abnormality of rate and represents the first indicators of respiratory distress (adults and children).

**Bradypnoea** – lower than the normal rate, includes disorders that cause Central Nervous System depression e.g. opiates, fatigue, severe hypoxia, hypothermia.

**Note** Children have a limited ability to increase pulmonary functional residual capacity, hence, increase their ventilation primarily by an increased respiratory rate rather than taking deeper breaths.

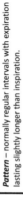

**Pattern** – normally regular intervals with expiration lasting slightly longer than inspiration.

Causes of altered patterns of breathing are Kussmaul's respiration (Diabetic Ketoacidosis); Cheyne-Stokes respiration (marked hypoxaemia).

**Depth** (tidal volume). Chest movements may be difficult to view in a patient with quiet shallow breathing, particularly when unconscious, and on its own is a subjective and inaccurate assessment. Note whether the patient is breathing deeply or shallow. If unsure, place a hand on their chest and gauge how far it rises and falls. Little movement indicates 'shallow' breathing.

A spirometer is the most accurate way of measurement (tidal volume). The normal tidal volume for an 'average' adult is 500mls and for a school aged child is 8–10 ml/kg. For the infant and small child this is 5–8 ml/kg.

**FIGURE 2.6** Respiratory assessment

# RESPIRATORY ASSESSMENT 2

**Procedure for measuring tidal volume using a spirometer**

- Explain procedure and gain consent.
- Wash and dry hands before and after procedure.
- Patient should breathe normally into the tube.
- Do not instruct the patient to take a deep breath, as a deep breath will falsely increase the results.
- Read the dial. Take the best result out of three.

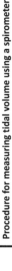

***Work of breathing*** – indicates degree of difficulty in breathing. Observe for use of accessory muscles (sternocleidomastoid, scalene and trapezius). Skin will become cool and clammy.

**Note** – An inability to talk in complete sentences (staccato speech) is a sign of severe respiratory distress.

In children nasal flaring and mouth breathing are common indicators. Increased respiratory rate, shoulders rising on inspiration, head bobbing with intercostal retractions indicate respiratory distress.

A baby normally uses their abdominal muscles to breathe and a school aged child uses their costal muscles for breathing. Respiratory distress should be suspected in a baby who uses its costal muscles and a child using its abdominal muscles to breathe.

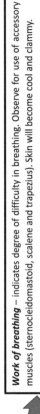

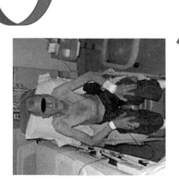

*Posture* - a 'tripod' position is adopted by those with respiratory impairment.

**FIGURE 2.7** Respiratory assessment 2

# RESPIRATORY ASSESSMENT 3

**Skin colour** – can be difficult to detect and particularly with dark skin. Observe for peripheral (nail beds, fingertips and toes) and central (lips, nose, mucous membrane of the mouth and tongue) cyanosis. Central cyanosis is a late clinical sign of respiratory problems.

**Symmetry of chest movement** – chest should move bilateral and equal, expanding on inspiration and expiration. If this cannot be seen clearly, stand in front of the patient with both hands firmly placed on each side of the anterior thorax so that equal expansion of the chest wall can be assessed.

**Pain** – of any origin can influence the patient's ability to breathe properly (reducing tidal volume). Pleuritic pain can be sharp/stabbing / localized pain, worst when breathing in deeply or coughing. Retention of sputum may occur resulting in possible atelectasis.
Assessment of pain in a child should be performed using an appropriate assessment pain tool, depending on the child's age and stage of development together with the use of play.

**Chest deformities** – may include a 'barrel' shape, kyphosis or scoliosis, all interfering with lung expansion.
Nail clubbing and swelling of the terminal part of the digit of fingertips/toes, nail thinning and an abnormal alteration in the angle of the finger/toes are indicative of chronic pulmonary or cardiovascular disease.

**Cough**
- Regularity.
- Presence or absence of pain.
- Distinctive sounds (e.g. whoop or bark, bubbling).
- Strength of cough.
- Is the cough unproductive (dry and/or 'tickly') or productive (producing sputum)?
- Secretions.
- Degree of breathlessness after coughing.
- Changes of colour to face during coughing (may become blue, red, very pale).

**Sputum**
- **White, frothy, pink** (bloodstained) – may indicate pulmonary oedema.
- **Frank blood** (haemoptysis) – possible pulmonary embolism or active tuberculosis (TB).
- **Blood stained** (streaks) – could imply pneumonia, abscess, aspiration (stomach contents).
- **Purulent Green** and copious – usually suggests infection.
- **Black** (tar) – usually old blood from very heavy smoking or industrial – e.g. mining job.
- **Rusty/brown** – may be a sign of Tuberculosis (TB), lung cancer.

**Mental status** – assess for signs of hypoxaemia (reduced level of consciousness). In babies, assessment could include recognition of a familiar voice, carer's face, favourite toy. Young children who can vocalise, can be asked the above questions, using simple, age appropriate language. Ask parents/carer for their conclusions of the child's mental status. Be mindful of language barriers/cultural barriers.

**FIGURE 2.8** Respiratory assessment 3

**Activity: now test yourself**

1. List five factors that influence pulse rate.

2. **True** or **false**? A child's blood pressure varies with age and is closely related to their height and weight.

3. List five factors influencing blood pressure.

4. What is the most accurate way to take a temperature? What potential dangers are associated with this route?

5. A tripod position involves the patient:

   a) sitting upright, leaning forward with hands supported by knees

   b) sitting upright, leaning forward with hands supported by knees, use of accessory muscles, pursed lips

   c) sitting upright, leaning forward, use of accessory muscles

   d) leaning forward, pursed lips

## Answers

1. Any of the following:

   Tachycardia:

   - emotion (stimulation of sympathetic nerve plus adrenaline)
   - exercise (epinephrine and lactic acid release)
   - drugs (bronchodilators, thyroxine, amphetamines)
   - temperature (metabolic rate increased)
   - shock (vasoconstriction)
   - hypoxaemia (initial increased sympathetic activity).

   Bradycardia:

   - cardiac dysrhythmias (sinoatrial or atrialventricular nodes)
   - hypothermia (decreased sinoatrial node impulses)
   - nervous system disorders/neurological insult (impairs control of autonomic nervous system)
   - drugs (e.g. beta-blockers).

2. True.

3. Any of the following:

   - a weak contraction of the heart (reduced cardiac output)
   - systemic vascular resistance (vasoconstriction as seen in shock)
   - disease process (e.g. arteriosclerosis)
   - blood volume (hypovolaemia/reduced preload); fluid retention (causing hypertension)
   - anxiety/stress/emotions/pain (catecholamine release)
   - diet (increased salt, alcohol and caffeine)

- ethnicity (hypertension linked to Afro–Caribbean and Asian origins)

- drugs (e.g. Ibuprofen increases/diuretics decrease blood pressure)

- gender (premenopausal women have a lower blood pressure than men of the same age; postmenopausal woman have a higher blood pressure)

- age (blood pressure gradually increases with age)

- diurnal variations (peaks in the late afternoon/evening and is at its lowest in the early hours of the morning during deep sleep)

- incorrect equipment

- incorrect technique.

4. Rectal temperature as this is closest to the body's core. Not routinely performed on children – risk of perforation and very traumatising psychologically. Stimulation of vagus nerve can cause cardiac arrhythmias.

5. a) sitting upright, leaning forward with hands supported by knees.

## Reflection: ask yourself

1. What do I know now that I didn't know before?

2. What am I confused/unclear about?

3. What areas do I need to focus on?

4. My action plan for further learning (make objectives SMART – Specific/Measurable/Achievable/Realistic/Time-bound):

# CHAPTER 3

# Oxygenation

Tina Moore

## Overview

There is no dispute that adequate oxygenation is essential for sustained life. Changes in the patient's respiratory status is one of the early warning signs of physiological deterioration, although a significant number of nurses state that changes in respiratory status is the least important indicator of patient deterioration (Mok et al., 2015). If changes are identified early, this may influence the outcome for patients.

### Link to *Future Nurse Proficiencies* (NMC 2018)

*Platform 3* Assessing needs and planning care (Sections 3.2; 3.4; 3.5).

**Annexe B, Part 1**: Procedures for assessing people's needs for person-centred care. Specifically, 2.5: manage and interpret cardiac monitors, infusion pumps, blood glucose monitors and other monitoring devices and 2.6: accurately measure weight and height, calculate body mass index and recognise healthy ranges and clinically significant low/high readings.

**Annexe B, Part 2**: Procedures for the planning, provision and management of person-centred nursing care. Specifically, 3.5: take appropriate action to reduce or minimise pain or discomfort; and Section 8: use evidence-based, best practice approaches for meeting needs for respiratory care and support, accurately assessing the person's capacity for independence and self-care and initiating appropriate interventions. Specifically, 8.3: take and interpret peak flow and oximetry measurements and 8.5: manage inhalation, humidifier and nebuliser devices.

## Expected knowledge

- Anatomy and physiology in relation to the respiratory system
- Physiology of the transportation of oxygen
- Process of gaseous exchange
- Factors influencing optimal gaseous exchange
- Chapter 1, Anatomy and physiology of the cardiovascular and respiratory system.

## Introduction

Deterioration of the patient's respiratory status is one of the early warning signs of physiological deterioration. Subsequently, appropriate assessment and early, effective intervention is para-mount. There are various devices used to assess the adequacy of gaseous exchange (for example pulse oximetry); assess problems with oxygen intake (for example peak flow, but *not* if the patient is too breathless); and improve gas exchange/oxygenation of the tissues (for example, administration of oxygen).

The administration of oxygen is used in many practice settings, and is often the first line of treatment. Even today, experiences suggest that oxygen is often given without careful appraisal of its potential benefits and side effects, regularly delegated to junior staff and students. Inappropriate dosage and failure to monitor the effects of oxygen therapy can have serious consequences.

## Content

| Related physiology | Procedure for pulse oximetry and peak flow assessments | Devices for the administration of supplementary oxygen |
|---|---|---|
| Signs of hypoxaemia and related management | Procedure for the administration of oxygen therapy | Nebuliser therapy |

## Learning outcomes

- Appraise the causes and levels of hypoxaemia
- Identify reasons for oxygen saturation monitoring and its limitations
- Demonstrate knowledge, understanding and skill in the procedures for assessing oxygen saturation and peak flow
- Identify with rationale the correct device for oxygen therapy
- Recognise the need for and administer nebuliser therapy.

## Key background

For the treatment of hypoxaemia to be successful and also dictate the amount of supplementary oxygen to be given, it is important to identify the cause of the problem. Essentially, there are four stages in the transfer of oxygen to the cells. Each, if compromised, can contribute to hypoxaemia.

Stage 1 involves the movement of oxygen from the atmosphere into the alveoli. This is the mechanism of ventilation (mechanical movement of gas or air into and out of the lung, i.e. inspiration and expiration). Ventilation is usually an involuntary process and involves homeostatic changes that can adjust the breathing rate and volume automatically via the medulla oblongata in the brain stem to maintain adequate gaseous exchange. Chemoreceptors are also involved in this process. These are located in the circulatory system (carotid and aortic bodies) and medulla oblongata, and sense the effectiveness of ventilation by monitoring the pH status of the cerebrospinal fluid, oxygen content ($PaO_2$) and carbon dioxide ($PaCO_2$) content of the arterial blood gas (ABG). These respond to hypercapnia (high carbon dioxide levels), acidaemia (low pH levels) and hypoxaemia (low oxygen levels) by sending impulses to the medulla to alter the rate of ventilation. In chronic obstructive pulmonary disease (COPD) these receptors become insensitive to small changes in $PaCO_2$ and as a result the regulation of ventilation is poor, which means that this group of patients will have a higher than normal $PaCO_2$ level.

It is worth noting that ventilation is not the same as respiration. Respiration is the exchange of gases (oxygen and carbon dioxide) during cellular metabolism. **Here, management revolves around improving the flow of oxygen into the alveoli, e.g. by nebuliser therapy.**

Stage 2 is comprised of the diffusion and transfer of oxygen across the alveolar capillary membrane. Oxygen moves from an area of high pressure to an area of low pressure until equilibrium is achieved. This process is helped by a surfactant which is secreted by the alveolar cells and maintains its integrity by covering the inner surface of the alveolus and lowering alveolar surface tension at the end of expiration, thus preventing atelectasis.

Stage 3 is the transport of oxygen within the circulation via the haemoglobin molecule. As oxygen diffuses across the alveolar capillary membrane, it dissolves into the plasma where it exerts pressure. As the partial pressure of oxygen increases in the plasma, oxygen moves into the erythrocytes (red blood cells) and binds with haemoglobin until it becomes 'saturated'.

Measurement of haemoglobin concentration is important when assessing individuals with respiratory problems. This is because a decrease in haemoglobin concentration below the normal value of blood reduces PaO2. Increases in haemoglobin concentration may increase oxygen content, minimising the impact of impaired gas exchange. Respiratory disease impairs gas exchange and an adequate plasma level of PaO2 is essential for the remaining oxygen to bind with the haemoglobin in order to facilitate tissue perfusion. **For stages 2 and 3, management is focused upon improving gas exchange, e.g. Continuous Positive Airway Pressure (CPAP)/Non Invasive Ventilation (NIV).**

Stage 4, the final stage, is the movement of oxygen from the haemoglobin to the tissues/cells. This is done through a concentration gradient, from high concentration in the alveoli to lower concentrations in the capillaries. This process is influenced by haemoglobin (Hb) levels (a decrease will reduce oxygen content). This process continues until the haemoglobin binding sites are what is referred to as 'saturated', i.e. full of oxygen. **Optimising Hb levels – it is important that Hb levels are within normal range (or as much as possible).**

# PULSE OXIMETRY

**Hypoxaemia**

Normal PaO2 = 11.5–13.5 kPa.

Mild to moderate hypoxaemia (10.5–5.0 kPa) may cause malaise, light-headedness, vertigo, impaired judgement, confusion, tachypnoea, dyspnoea, tachycardia.

Severe hypoxaemia (PaO2 <4.5 kPa) may cause bradycardia, lethargy, oliguria, hypotension, diaphoresis central cyanosis. Eventually, coma, convulsions and possibly respiratory arrest. Note that cyanosis will NOT be present in patients with anaemia.

**Treatment for hypoxaemia**

Administration of oxygen alone will not help to prevent/alleviate hypoxaemia.

- Position should be upright where possible.
- Maintenance of adequate fluid balance/maintenance of adequate blood pressure (for sufficient delivery of oxygenated blood to the tissues).
- Slow, deep breaths (increases tidal volume, improving gaseous exchange).
- Physiotherapy if indicated.
- Supplementary oxygen as prescribed.
- Compliance is essential and is required continuously. Confusion may be a symptom of hypoxia.
- Non-invasive ventilation, if there is no response to the above.

Pulse oximetry monitoring offers simple, reliable and quick measurement of the oxygen saturation levels of peripheral capillary blood (SpO2). This should be analysed in the context of the amount of inspired oxygen that the patient is receiving and also as part of a full and comprehensive respiratory assessment.

Note that SpO2 monitoring does not provide a picture of the overall efficiency of gas exchange in the lungs or tissues, i.e. carbon dioxide levels (particularly important when determining deterioration). If indicated, ABG analysis should be performed together with comprehensive respiratory assessment.

Do **NOT** use on patients with carbon monoxide poisoning (the probe cannot differentiate between oxyhaemoglobin and carboxyhaemoglobin and will provide false high oxygen saturation (SpO2) readings).

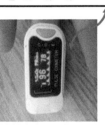

**Procedure for pulse oximetry monitoring**

1. Explain procedure and gain consent where possible.
2. Wash and dry hands before and after procedure.
3. Ensure the device is working (test it on yourself). Use the correct probe size. Usually finger is used. Follow manufactures guidance on where to place the probe (toe, earlobe).
4. Remove any dark coloured nail polish (e.g. black, blue), for close monitoring peripheral colour and capillary refill time.
5. Clean patient's skin (following manufacturer's guidelines, e.g. soap and water or alcohol impregnated swabs). Ensure skin is thoroughly dry. Attach well-fitting probe.
6. Avoid using the same arm as the blood pressure recordings. Alarm limits should be set for continuous monitoring (low saturation and high/low pulse rate). Normally these are automatically set to default values when the device is switched on i.e. oxygen saturation less than 95% (unless COPD – then 92%) (BTS, 2017).
7. Note that pulse volume, peripheral perfusion, direct sunlight and arrhythmias may affect amplitude.
8. Document findings.
9. Change probe position at least four-hourly, pressure sores and damage to the tissue by the heat expelled may occur.

**FIGURE 3.1** Pulse oximetry

# OXYGEN THERAPY (O2) 1

Oxygen (O2) therapy (unless an emergency situation) should always be prescribed. Have a target goal (oxygen saturation) for intervention. Despite receiving O2 therapy, the patient's condition may WORSEN.

**Low flow systems (variable performance systems)** depend upon the patient's minute ventilation, peak inspiratory flow rate and O2 flow rate. These can be variable throughout O2 administration. These systems do not always provide all the gas necessary to meet the patient's total minute ventilation requirements.

It is difficult to estimate **exactly** how much inspired O2 a patient is receiving. Devices include: simple face masks; nasal cannulae; partial re-breathing mask and non-rebreathing mask.

The concentration of O2 delivered is dependent upon the minute volume (breathing rate and tidal volume). If the patient has an increased minute volume the concentration of O2 delivered is decreased. Deep, slow breaths will cause a much higher concentration of O2 to be inspired.

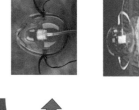

### Procedure of giving oxygen

1. Where possible, explain procedure and gain consent.
2. Select the correct device.
3. Note – masks may cause claustrophobia. You may need to let the patient get used to the mask first by placing and holding gently on their face for a few minutes.
4. Securely mask over mouth, nose and chin. Press the metal piece over the bridge of the nose firmly.
5. Adjust straps to fit correctly. You should be able to move two fingers inside the strap.
6. Young children may be frightened and agitated when O2 is administered and feel a sense of claustrophobia. A parent could hold the mask in proximity to or over the child's face instead.
7. Assess respiratory status and record O2 saturation levels at start of the administration and monitor accordingly.
8. Attach to humidifier for long term O2 therapy (over 24 hours). Check mask/tubing for accumulation of water and remove/wipe periodically. If heated, ensure it is not set too hot.
9. Document what is administered and what device.
10. Ensure patient has a sputum pot and tissues.
11. If safe and appropriate, patients should have the O2 via a nasal cannula during meal times.

**Simple face mask** – delivers up to 60% of diluted concentration of O2. For this device, O2 flow must be at least 5 l/min to prevent collection and rebreathing of exhaled gas.

**Partial rebreathing mask and bag** – a reservoir bag added to the face mask provides greater than 60% O2. Deflate the bag by only one third on inspiration (prevents accumulation of O2). High flow rates will cause drying and irritation of the eyes. Artificial eye drops may need to be prescribed.

**FIGURE 3.2** Oxygen therapy 1

# OXYGEN THERAPY (O2) 2

**Non-rebreathing bag and mask** provide high concentrations of O2 from a reservoir mask and are used for all patients who are critically ill. The flow rate should be at 10–15 litres. During inspiration the side port valves of the mask close and the valve between the bag and mask connection opens allowing for inspiration of approximately 100% O2. The opposite occurs during expiration. These valves are designed to prevent exhaled gas from entering the reservoir bag, eliminating rebreathing of expired gas.

The reservoir bag should not collapse during inspiration (suggesting flow rates are insufficient to meet the patient's ventilatory demands). If this occurs the patient may struggle against the one way valve and therefore work of breathing is increased leading to tiredness and exhaustion.

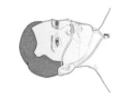

Nasal cannulae are simple and unobtrusive devices delivering a flow of O2 from 24%–44%. Up to 4 litres is the norm but flow rate can be as high as 6 litres (monitor for signs of epistaxis). Useful for patients unable to tolerate a mask or who are eating and drinking, coughing, expectorating copious amounts of sputum or vomiting. Only suitable for short term administration. This device is not effective for patients who are 'mouth breathers'. Inspect skin for pressure sores and nasal cavity from drying and irritation particularly if receiving humidified O2.

Inspect the nasal cavity and around the sides of the nose regularly for pressure sores. Place gauze padding around the ears between the patient's skin and tubing to minimise risk of pressure sores. Humidification can help with drying and irritation. Nasal care should be given with cotton buds.

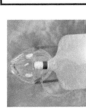

### High flow systems (fixed performance masks)

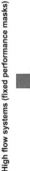

**Venturi Mask** allows for a fixed flow of O2. This is facilitated through a jet adapter that is positioned between the mask and tubing to the O2 source. O2 rates are set above the normal respiratory flow rate and are available in the following colour coded concentrations: 24%; 28%; 35%; 40% and 60%.

This device is best used for patients who require an accurate concentration of O2 (e.g. COPD), making blood gas analysis more meaningful.

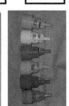

**FIGURE 3.3** Oxygen therapy 2

# PEAK FLOW METER

A peak flow meter is a small hand-held device that measures the 'peak expiratory flow' (PEF), and helps to assess the airflow through the airways (determining the degree of obstruction).

The low-range peak flow meter is used for small children (4–9 years) and adults with severely impaired lung function. The standard-range peak flow meter is used for older children, teenagers and adults.
Normal peak flow rates vary according to age, height, and sex. However, a patient's normal score should be within 20% of a person of the same age, sex, and height who does not have asthma.

## Procedure for recording peak flow

1. Explain procedure and the rationale for the skill. Gain consent.
2. Demonstrate the skill, giving clear instructions.
3. Sit patient in an upright position.
4. Wash and dry hands before and after the procedure.
5. The red cursor along the side of the device should be set at zero. Ensure that the hand is not touching the cursor as it will not move.
6. Place the disposable mouthpiece securely at the top of the device.
7. Hold peak flow meter horizontally in front of the mouth. Instruct the patient to take a deep breath on inspiration, close the lips firmly around the mouthpiece, ensuring there is no air leak around the lips.
8. Patient should then breathe out as hard and as fast as possible.
9. Where the cursor stops should be noted.
10. Return cursor to zero and instruct the patient to repeat this sequence twice more (total of three readings).
11. The highest score of all three measurements should be recorded.
12. Remove and discard the disposable mouthpiece.
13. Document results.

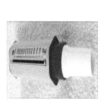

Peak flow meter

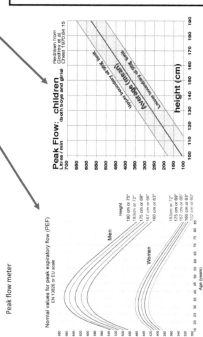

Peak Flow: children
both boys and girls
Litres / min

Average (mean)
Lower boundary of peak flow
Upper boundary of peak flow

height (cm)

Redrawn from
Godfrey et al.
Chest 1970;84:15

Normal peak flow values for children

Normal values for peak expiratory flow (PEF)
EN 13826 or EU scale

Height

Men

Women

Age (years)

PEF (L/min)

Normal peak flow values for adults

**FIGURE 3.4** Peak flow meter (PERF)

# NEBULISER THERAPY

## Procedure for administering nebuliser treatments

1. Explain the procedure and gain consent. Explain possible side effects of the medication e.g. tremor, tachycardia, dizziness, dry mouth, irritation to the eyes.
2. Wash hands before and after the procedure.
3. Where appropriate, sit patient upright and teach and encourage deep breathing and to cough after administration. Provide sputum pot and tissues.
4. If appropriate, take a peak flow reading before administration.
5. Open storage chamber of the mask and insert the solution, reattach the storage chamber. Ensure the attachments are secure.
6. Normally air (via a cylinder) is used. Note – that a fine spray/mist and a hissing sound will occur if done correctly and the flow is high enough. Oxygen can be used as the driving gas but caution is required for patients with COPD.
7. Note, if the patient is severely hypoxaemic, supplementary oxygen may be prescribed during nebuliser therapy (via a nasal cannula). Monitor respiratory status closely.
8. Check the device is working first before attaching the mask to the patient. For the child/patient who feels claustrophobic and those patients who are very anxious, let them feel the moisture/steam first by putting the mask gently next to their face. Do not apply the straps of the mask yet. Once they have got used to it then gently strap the mask. Divisional therapy / play may also be required.
9. Monitoring of oxygen saturation throughout this procedure if appropriate.
10. A gas flow rate of 6-8 litres is required. Stop once storage chamber is empty (there may be a little residue left in the chamber). Time for administration is generally 7-10 minutes.
11. Measure post nebuliser peak flow (normally after 30 minutes).
12. Any residue should be discarded and the nebuliser mask and storage chamber should be washed, dried and placed by the patient's bedside for future usage.
13. Observe patient's eyes (mist/moisture may cause some irritation).
14. Document findings/administration.

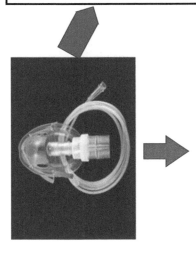

**Nebuliser devices** administer drugs via inhalation, mainly bronchodilators, mucolytics, corticosteroids or antibiotics for lower respiratory tract problems. Normally nebulized treatment is given via air, but can be delivered through oxygen if the patient has moderate to severe hypoxaemia. Constant observations are required for signs of hyperoxia.

The cylinder should have a minimum flow rate of 6-8l/min. Once the nebulizer therapy is complete, the patient should be changed back to their usual device. If necessary, supplementary oxygen should also be give (concurrently) by nasal cannulae at 2-4 l/min in an attempt to maintain an oxygen saturation levels.

**FIGURE 3.5** Nebuliser therapy

## Activity: now test yourself

1. List four symptoms of mild hypoxaemia and four symptoms of severe hypoxaemia.

   **True** or **false**? Pulse oximetry provides information about oxygen saturation levels and carbon dioxide levels.

3. Low flow oxygen delivery systems are:

   a) variable performance systems and allow for the calculation of the exact amount of oxygen delivered to the patient

   b) fixed performance systems and are useful for patients who require precise levels of oxygen delivery

   c) variable performance systems and are dependent upon the patient's minute volume, peak inspiratory flow rate and oxygen flow rate

   d) venturi masks, non-rebreathing bag and mask.

4. When would you use a peak flow meter to assess the patients respiratory status?

5. Nebuliser devices:

   a) provide the administration of drugs via inhalation

   b) can be given concurrently with oxygen therapy

   c) require, in their administration, constant observation for side effects of the drugs used

   d) all of the above.

**Answers**

1. Any of the following:

   Mild hypoxaemia:

   *Malaise, light headedness, dizziness, vertigo, confusion, impaired judgement, tachypnoea, dyspnoea, tachycardia*

   Severe hypoxaemia

   *Lethargy, hypotension, oliguria, bradycardia, central cyanosis, coma, respiratory arrest, diaphoresis, seizures*

2. False.

   *This is one of the largest limitations of pulse oximetry monitoring. So, if there are concerns regarding the patient's rising carbon dioxide levels, an ABG should be performed and the results analysed.*

3. c) low flow oxygen delivery systems are variable performance systems and are dependent upon the patient's minute volume, peak inspiratory flow rate and oxygen flow rate.

4. A peak flow meter measures the peak expiratory flow, providing information about the patient's airflow through their airways, particularly bronchi; a low reading will normally indicate possible air trapping and compromised gaseous exchange. This usually is performed on people with asthma and COPD or any patient that may have obstruction to their airflow. Peak flow readings may drop before the patient starts to wheeze or cough: if patients are dyspnoeic or breathless it may be unsafe to use this as part of your assessment.

5. d) all of the above.

## Reflection: ask yourself

1. What do I know now that I didn't know before?

2. What am I confused/unclear about?

3. What areas do I need to focus on?

4. My action plan for further learning (make objectives SMART – Specific/Measurable/Achievable/Realistic/Time-bound):

# CHAPTER 4

# Advanced respiratory skills

*Tina Moore*

## Overview

Respiratory disorders are commonly experienced by patients. This can be due to primary causes (e.g. asthma, COPD, pneumonia) or secondary (e.g. heart failure). So as a student nurse you will care for a patient with a respiratory disorder. During events of acute illness and/or physiological deterioration compensatory changes to the respiratory system occur early. Therefore the respiratory rate is one of the early warning signs. As a result, student nurses will also be involved in the care management of patients with respiratory disorders.

### Link to *Future Nurse Proficiencies* (NMC 2018)

**Platform 3** Assessing needs and planning care (Sections 3.1; 3.2; 3.5).

**Platform 4** Providing and evaluating care (Sections 4.1; 4.3; 4.5; 4.12).

**Annexe B, Part 1**: Procedures for assessing people's needs for person-centred care. Specifically, 2.8: undertake chest auscultation and interpret findings and 2.13: identify and respond to signs of deterioration and sepsis.

**Annexe B, Part 2**: Use evidence-based, best practice approaches for meeting needs for respiratory care and support, accurately assessing the person's capacity for independence and self-care and initiating appropriate interventions. Specifically, 8.4: use appropriate nasal and oral suctioning techniques and 8.6: manage airway and respiratory processes and equipment.

## Expected knowledge

* Anatomy and physiology of the upper and lower respiratory systems, gas exchange
* Anatomy of the pleura
* Causes and signs of hypoxaemia
* Correct use of stethoscope
* Chapter 1, Anatomy and physiology of the respiratory system.

## Introduction

There are many patients whose condition will be/is at risk of deterioration and where early warning signs are triggered. The deterioration is sometimes unpredictable. It is essential to remember that not all patients will provide 'early warning signs' of deterioration, often making it impossible for prediction to occur. For most of these patients, the monitoring of fundamental vital signs alone will be insufficient to detect significant physiological changes. In effect, the more intricate the patient's condition is, the more complex the methods of assessment and management knowledge and skills must be.

Signs of respiratory failure include:

* Respiratory compensation (tachypnoea, use of accessory muscles, nasal flaring, suprasternal recession in children)
* Increased sympathetic tone (tachycardia, hypertension, sweating)
* Hypoxia (confusion, agitation, disorientation (bradycardia, coma in late stages)
* Haemoglobin desaturation (cyanosis, low oxygen saturation levels, acid base imbalances).

## Content

| Indications for and types of tracheostomies | Types of tracheostomy tubes | Management of a tracheostomy tube including suctioning |
|---|---|---|
| Procedure for lung auscultation | Basic lung sounds | Reasons for ABG analysis |
| Obtaining arterial blood sample | Acid base imbalances | Management of chest drain including removal |

## Learning outcomes

- Demonstrate knowledge and understanding of a tracheostomy and the appropriate use of the different types of tracheostomy tubes
- Use the correct techniques and plan of care to provide safe and appropriate tracheostomy care
- Describe and interpret normal and abnormal lung sounds
- Be able to interpret arterial blood gas analysis
- Manage the care of a patient with an insertion of a chest drain.

## Key background

There are many advanced skills that were traditionally carried out by medical staff only. But with additional training, experience and assessment, other health care professionals including nurses can perform these functions.

Lung auscultation (direct or indirect) is a non-invasive method of listening to lung sounds. This should be part of any comprehensive respiratory assessment. It is important to listen to each lung sound independently, right (apex, midzone and base) and left (apex and base). There should be a description of what is heard. It is important to determine between normal, abnormal and additional lung sounds.

Whilst pulse oximetry monitoring is advantageous in that it is non-invasive and can provide a quick summary of the patient's oxygenation status, it does not provide all the information required particularly for those patients who are acutely/critically ill or deteriorating. In these scenarios, the ventilatory status of the patient (namely, carbon dioxide levels) are extremely important. Therefore, there will be instances when arterial blood from the patient is required for a higher level assessment of the patient's respiratory (and/or metabolic) status. This is in the form of arterial blood gas monitoring.

The point cannot be stressed enough that it is the responsibility of those in charge to ensure that assessment and care management is performed by someone suitably qualified, knowledgeable, competent and skilful.

It cannot be emphasised enough that it is imperative to analyse the observation data in the context of what is considered to be the patient's normal parameters. Particularly in the instance of long-term conditions where there have been a period of years during which the patient has adapted and adjusted to their condition, 'abnormal' parameters can become their 'normal'. For example, oxygen saturation levels in Chronic Obstructive Pulmonary Disorder (COPD).

# TRACHEOSTOMY

## Main types of tracheostomies

*Cricothyoidotomy* (mini tracheostomy) – an opening in the cricoid membrane allowing quick safe access to the airway for emergency or difficult intubations. A cuffless tracheostomy tube is used. This can also be used for an oxygenation and suctioning purposes. A more difficult procedure in children.

*Percutaneous tracheostomy* – more common. As a dilator is used, it is easier, safer and faster than a surgical procedure.

## Indications for a Tracheostomy

*To reduce work of breathing* – there is up to 50% reduction in the 'anatomical dead space', improving gas exchange.

*Endotracheal intubation* lasting more than 2 weeks can result in tracheal stenosis.

*Bypass severe acute upper airway obstruction* (e.g. foreign body; severe upper airway infections; burns, swelling)

Remove of excessive bronchial secretions

## Cuffed tracheostomy tube

Normally used in Critical Care areas and not recommended for children. Cuffed tubes allow for positive pressure ventilation and help to prevent aspiration. Patients cannot eat or drink (unless balloon is deflated).

Cuff pressure should be between 20–25 cm $H_2O$ (ICS, 2014) otherwise irritation and tracheal wall damage can occur. Measure a minimum of once every 8 hours with pressure manometer.

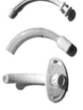
Cuffed tracheostomy tube

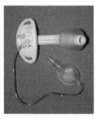
Non fenestrated (uncuffed) tube

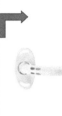
Manometer

## Non fenestrated (uncuffed) tubes

Most tubes have an outer and inner (removable) tube. The outer cannula is passed into the trachea (size usually refers to the inner diameter of the outer cannula). The inner cannula has the standard 15mm attachment that connects to oxygen etc. Failure to properly lock the inner tube in place can unlock the inner cannula in some devices resulting in disconnection of the breathing circuit (in circumstances where it is connected to this rather than the outer cannula). **Single-lumen tubes have no inner cannula.**

The first outer tube is usually changed 5–7 days post insertion. The inner tube enables an open airway (from occlusion caused by mucus). Removing just the inner tube may be enough to clear secretions can provide immediate relief of life-threatening airway obstruction in the event of blockage of a tracheostomy tube with blood clot or encrusted secretions.

Maximum intervals for removing and cleaning inner tubes are recommended as four-hourly for patients with a productive cough and eight-hourly for other patients (ICS 2014). The inner tube should be cleaned with sterile water or 0.9% saline.

## Fenestrated tubes

Fenestrated tubes have single or multiple 'holes', permitting airflow, allowing the patient to talk and cough more effectively. Patients must sit upright to minimise the risk of aspiration.

Cuffed fenestrated tubes can be used during the weaning process. Uncuffed tubes are used when patients no longer depend on a cuffed tube and are not at risk of aspiration. Do NOT suction through a fenestrated tube, change the inner tube to non-fenestrated.

**FIGURE 4.1** Indications for and types of tracheostomies

# TRACHEOSTOMY CARE

In the instance of any infectious situation, follow national and local guidelines in relation to the use of personal protective equipment and procedures.

**Emergency equipment**

At the bedside and should be checked at least once per shift:

- Tracheal dilators
- Suction machine/appropriate size catheters
- Disposable gloves/apron
- Goggles (follow Trust policy)
- Oxygen with tracheostomy mask
- 10ml syringe (if cuffed)
- Scissors/stitch cutter (if tube is stitched in)
- Non rebreathing bag and tubing and/or bag-valve mask with reservoir and tubing
- Tracheostomy tubes – one same size and one size smaller

**Dressing**

Following surgery, leave original dressing for first 48 hours (change only if the dressing is soiled). Aseptically clean stoma with 0.9% saline at least once every 24 hours. Swab if stoma is sore and red. Do not cream the area unless prescribed.

During first few days, risk of tube displacement is very high. Generally sutures are not used, instead the tube is kept in place by cotton tapes through the neck plate. TWO people are required to change the dressing/tapes (holding the tube and the other performing the dressing).

**Humidification**

Life-threatening blockage can occur without humidification e.g. tenacious sputum, keratinisation and ulceration of the tracheal mucosa. Leading to sputum retention and impaired gaseous exchange.

Physiotherapy, early patient mobilisation, adequate hydration, appropriate suctioning, prompt treatment of infection, mucolytics saline nebulizers may be required.

Heated devices may be indicated. Infection can occur from the condensation, follow hospital and manufacturer's guidance to prevent this.

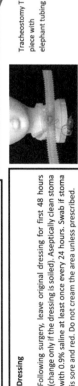

Tracheostomy T piece with elephant tubing

Tracheostomy oxygen mask

***Blocked tracheostomy tube***

The most serious complication and is a life threatening emergency.

Humidification is used to minimise risk, ensure cleanliness and patency of the inner tube by changing it as per guidelines, secure fixation of the tube and maintain correct cuff pressure.

- Assess urgency – contact anaesthetist immediately.
- Encourage patient to cough if possible.
- Suction tracheostomy tube and oral pharynx.
- Alter position.
- Remove inner tube if present.
- If cuff inflated – deflate it and suction again by deflating the tube. This can also allow some air to get into the lungs.
- Remove tube and replace with spare tube.
- Give 100% oxygen.
- Monitor patient's respiratory status.
- Cardiac arrest call if patient has stopped breathing.

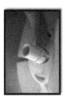

Neck plate

**FIGURE 4.2** Tracheostomy care

# SUCTIONING

**Procedure**

- Suctioning as an when indicated. Explain procedure and gain consent (play with child).
- NOTE – inner tube should be NON-FENESTRATED (prevents catheter from passing through the holes).
- Aseptic procedure. Equipment required = suction machine/suction catheters/sterile water for irrigation/clean disposable apron and gloves/sterile disposable container/bactericidal hand rub/goggles (Trust policy guidance)/sterile container.
- Sit patient upright with head and neck supported where possible.
- Wash and dry hands before and after the procedure.
- Check that the suction machine is on and working.
- Set at appropriate negative suction pressure (adult: 100–120 mmHg, child: 80–100mmHg, infants: 60–80 mmHg).
- Calculate appropriate catheter size – no larger than one half of the tube diameter. Suction catheter size (Fg) = 2 x (size of tracheostomy tube - 2).
- Hyperoxygenation and hyperinflation (take 5 deep breaths) prior to suctioning may be indicated. Repeat post suctioning. Any increase in oxygen should be prescribed by the doctor.
- Clean hands with alcohol rubs. Put on gloves.
- Withdraw catheter from sleeve without contaminating it.
- Insert the suction catheter. DO NOT apply negative pressure on insertion.
- On withdrawing the catheter slowly apply suction pressure (place thumb over suction port control).
- Withdraw catheter gently. No need to rotate with multiple-eyed (hole) catheters. Insertion and withdrawal should not take longer than 10–15 seconds.
- Monitor oxygen saturation and heart rate (may decrease with hypoxemia).
- On completion wrap catheter around gloved hand, pull back glove over soiled catheter and discard safely.
- Dip end of connection in jug of sterile water and discard other glove.
- Clean hands with bactericidal alcohol hand rub.
- If additional suctioning, start the procedure again with another catheter and glove.
- Repeat until the airway is clear (auscultate post suctioning). A maximum of three suction passes are suggested (Glass and Grap, 1995). Allow patient to rest between each suction pass.
- Reconnect oxygen as soon as possible.
- Ensure patient is left as comfortable as possible.
- Monitor for signs of infection, haemorrhage, atelectasis, prolonged cough.

Non disposable inner cannulae should be cleaned as required and according to the manufacturers' instructions or with sterile water and air dried thoroughly before replacing. Due to the risk of damage to the inner surface of the inner cannula we suggest that this should not be cleaned with a brush.

**FIGURE 4.3** Suctioning

# SPEAKING VALVE

## Speaking

Encourage patient to speak as soon as indicated. Speech and language therapist should be involved (particularly with children). Sound production occurs with fenestrated tubes. Cuffed tubes should only be used if the patient can tolerate the passive closure of the tracheostomy and as soon as the cuff can be deflated, a speaking valve can be used to enable to patient to speak and eat. This is a one-way valve fitting at the end of the tracheostomy tube.

Speaking valves allow patients to breathe in through the tracheostomy but NOT out and therefore can be extremely dangerous. Airflow has to go up through the larynx and out of the mouth, allowing the patient to talk (due to increased airflow resistance can be tiring). Speaking valves should ideally only be used with an un-cuffed and fenestrated tube (with fenestrated inner cannula).

Note – with the speaking valve in place the cuff must ALWAYS be deflated otherwise the patient cannot exhale and will asphyxiate, suffer barotrauma or lose cardiac output as intrathoracic pressure rises.

## Swallowing

Before eating and drinking, patients should be risk assessed for aspiration. Patients may also be referred to the Speech and Language Therapy Team (SALT). When able to swallow, start with sips of water. If no signs of respiratory distress (coughing, desaturation, increased tracheal secretions, increased respiratory rate) gradually increasing to free fluids and then soft diet.

Warn patient that initially they may feel discomfort on swallowing. Monitor fluid and nutritional intake, supplementing any deficit.

Speaking valve

**FIGURE 4.4** Speaking valve for tracheostomy

# LUNG AUSCULTATION

Assessment of breath sounds (with and without a stethoscope) should form part of the respiratory assessment. Indirect auscultation (with stethoscope) is a procedure undertaken by experienced practitioners who should have undergone appropriate training and education.

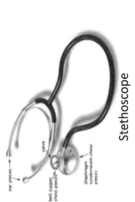

Stethoscope

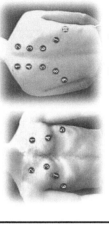

Main auscultation landmarks

Anterior      Posterior

**Procedure**

➤ Inform patient of procedure and gain consent where possible. Ensure privacy and dignity. Wash and dry hands before and after procedure. Ensure environment is not cold and is a quiet as possible.

➤ If possible place patient in an upright, leaning forward position. Expose chest and ensure that the stethoscope is not placed on clothing and dressings. Shaving of the chest may be necessary (too much hair can interfere with sound transmission). Gain consent before shaving.

➤ For children, play using the stethoscope will likely to be required in addition to distraction.

➤ The flat diaphragm is normally used for identifying high pitched sounds and the bell for low and medium frequency sounds.

➤ The tubing should be 48 cm (shorter tubing reduces further background noise). Ensure no kinks in the tubing.

➤ The patient should take slow deep breaths. Listen in an ordered sequence (landmarks) listening to the main areas, i.e. apex, midzone, base, anterior and posterior of right and left lung.

➤ Check audible by tapping the diaphragm.

➤ Close your eyes in order to try and block visual senses.

➤ Listen to inspiration and expiration separately on the anterior wall of the chest and then the posterior wall. Describe what is heard, i.e. frequency, pitch, intensity, duration and quality, are breath sounds clear, decreased or absent, and location of any adventitious (extra) sounds.

➤ Document whether the sound is heard direct (without stethoscope) or indirect (with stethoscope), compare each side to the other, when and where sounds are heard inspiratory or expiratory, cleared on coughing. These sounds can either be direct (sounds audible without a stethoscope) or indirect (use of stethoscope). Normally breathing should not be heard without the use of a stethoscope.

➤ Clean the stethoscope between uses (infection control) with different patients or by different members of staff (ideally all staff should have their own).

**FIGURE 4.5** Lung auscultation

# LUNG SOUNDS

## Normal:

Normal breathing should be quiet. Normal lung sounds are known as vesicular, bronchovesicuar and bronchial.

*Vesicular* sounds (low pitched, low intensity – described as 'soft and breezy') can be heard over most of the lung fields. In normal breathing, air moves into the airway during **inspiration** branching into progressively smaller and smaller airways as it moves to the alveoli. Turbulence of the airway which produces the sound (like wind rushing through trees – gentle 'swishing' sound). During **expiration**, air is flowing from small airways to much larger ones, and while the air does contact some surfaces, it takes place in larger, less confining tubes. Therefore, less turbulence created and less sound (as a smooth, swishing sound).

*Harsh Vesicular Breath Sound* – Much louder sounds occurring in conditions where breathing is rapid, producing deep breaths that are longer and louder breaths (faster and deeper breathing).

*Diminished Vesicular Breath Sound* – Softer, more distant in sound and can occur in the chest of someone who doesn't move as much air (i.e. shallow breathing).

*Bronchovesicular* sounds should be heard in the anterior region, near the mainstem bronchi and posterior only between the scapulae; sounds are more moderate in pitch and intensity. Heard equally throughout inspiration and expiration. There is no silent gap.

*Bronchial* sounds are high pitched, loud and hollow sounding and are normally heard over the larger airways and the trachea. They are course, loud, harsh sounds in which expiration is the predominant phase, usually heard throughout the whole of expiration and through only part of inspiration. If bronchial sounds are heard in other areas this could indicate consolidation of lung tissue, e.g. in pneumonia (consolidated lung tissue transmits sounds better than air, making it louder). There is also a silent gap between inspiration and expiration.

## Abnormal breath sounds

*Absent Breath Sounds* – may be localised, while the rest of the lung is normal or generalised indicating:

- Pneumothorax.
- Pleural effusion.
- Massive atelectasis (collapsed alveoli).
- Complete airway obstruction.

### Adventitious (additional) sounds:

*Crackles (rales)* – discontinuous, non-musical, breath sounds heard more commonly on inspiration and indicative of small airway disease (alveoli) and pulmonary oedema. Small airways open during inspiration and collapse during expiration causing the cracking (popping) sounds. When listening pay special attention to their loudness, pitch, duration, number, timing in the respiratory cycle, location, pattern from breath to breath, change after a cough or shift in position.

They can be classified as:

Fine crackles – high pitched and heard at the lung base near the end of inspiration.

Medium crackles – lower in pitch and heard during the middle/latter part of inspiration.

Course crackles – loud, bubbling sounds heard on both inspiration and expiration. Usually associated with mucous which may clear after coughing. If uncleaned, suctioning may be necessary.

*Rhonchi* – similar to wheezing but produces a continuous, bubbling, **gurgling low-pitched sound**. Heard most frequently during expiration. Indicates large airway disease. There are three categories:

Bubbling Rhonchi – secretions that are moving through the large bronchioles and bronchi. Can occur following surgery, pneumonia, overdose or on prolonged bed rest.

Gurgling Rhonchi – sounds heard throughout inspiration and expiration.

Sonorous Rhonchi – sounds similar to wheezing but has a low pitch sound. Heard more during expiration.

*Wheeze* – high pitched, squeaking, musical, continuous noises, mainly heard during expiration but can also be heard during inspiration. Indicative of constriction of the larger airways. Wheezes are classified in accordance with their severity:

Mild wheeze – seen in patients with some secretions.

Moderate wheeze – sounds for most of the expiratory phase.

Severe wheeze – occurs throughout the whole of inspiration and expiration.

**FIGURE 4.6** Lung sounds

# OBTAINING AN ARTERIAL BLOOD GAS (ABG) SAMPLE

ABG analysis is more accurate in assessing the efficiency of gas exchange (oxygenation and ventilation). This procedure is usually undertaken when the patient's condition is severe enough to warrant more detailed analysis, particularly of carbon dioxide levels. The technique is not only risky (bleeding, infection) but also extremely painful.

**Obtaining a sample**

Two routes used, an arterial line or an arterial stab (normally radial or femoral). Radial artery is usually selected as it is superficial, and easier to palpate, stabilise and puncture. The radial artery also has a collateral blood flow, so if damage or obstruction occurs the ulnar artery will maintain blood flow to the tissues. Collateral blood flow is confirmed by the Allen test. With peripheral shutdown or the radial artery cannot be palpated, the femoral artery may be used. But the risk of bleeding is greater. If regular ABG analysis is required, an arterial line should be inserted.

**Reasons for ABG analysis**

- Diagnosis and severity of respiratory failure
- Evaluate interventions (e.g. fluid resuscitation)
- Managing the acutely/critically ill (assessment of respiratory or metabolic disorders e.g. diabetic ketoacidosis, respiratory failure)
- Assess patient's condition immediately following cardio-pulmonary resuscitation
- Establish baseline for surgery
- Post 20 minutes of altering supplementary oxygen therapy
- Determine prognosis in the critically ill

- Pre-prepared syringes 0.5–1 ml for aspirating blood (adult) and 0.1–0.2 ml (child).
- Record blood taken each time on fluid balance chart, particularly for the child.
- Ensure no air bubbles are in the syringe (large air bubbles falsely increase the PaO2 content and reduce the PaCO2).
- Note the position of the patient, the supine position can cause a false reduction in PaO2. Where possible an upright position is best for this procedure.
- There is a high risk of bleeding. Once the needle has been withdrawn from the artery, apply continuous pressure for at least five minutes (longer if the patient has haematological problems or high risk of bleeding).
- Observe closely for signs of ischaemia, obstruction and nerve trauma (pins and needles, numbness, loss of wrist/hand movement).
- Once blood has been taken, the syringe should NOT be shaken vigorously, as this leads to haemolysis, gentle rolling is sufficient. Results should be analysed within 15 minutes at room temperature or the cells will start to metabolise in the syringe (using oxygen). Thus increasing PaCO2 and reducing PaO2.

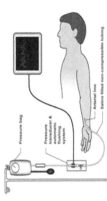

Pressure bag

Pressure transducer & automatic flushing system

Arterial line

Saline filled non-compressable tubing

Arterial line

**FIGURE 4.7** Obtaining arterial blood gas (ABG) samples

# INTERPRETING ARTERIAL BLOOD GAS (ABG) 1

**Acid base balance**

**pH** – measures blood acidity or alkalinity and provides information regarding the acid base balance. In absolute chemical terms pH is on a scale between 0 (absolute acid) to 14 (absolute alkaline).

Normal pH range for human blood normal range is 7.35–7.45 (alkaline). It is measured in moles per litre. Small changes in pH are life threatening.

The normal by product of cellular metabolism is carbon dioxide ($CO_2$). $CO_2$ is excreted by the lungs. Any excess combines with water ($H_2O$) to form carbon acid ($H_2CO_3$) (a weak acid). The pH changes in accordance to the amount of $H_2CO_3$ present. So, pH is inversely proportional to the number of hydrogen ions (H+) in the blood – as H+ accumulates, pH reduces. The kidneys reabsorb $H_2CO_3$ (to increase pH) and excrete hydrogen ions (to decrease pH).

Blood pH below 7.35 (acidotic) and pH above 7.45 (alkalotic).

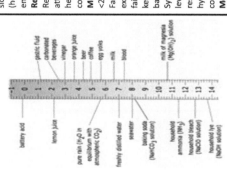

pH scale

**Respiratory acidosis** (pH <7.35mmol/l $PaCO_2$ >6.0kPa). Results from hypoventilation (inability to excrete $CO_2$). Causes include any condition where breathing becomes slower and shallow e.g. central nervous system depression (head injury), excessive use of sedatives, massive pulmonary embolism, pulmonary oedema, pneumonia.

**Respiratory alkalosis** (pH >7.45mmol/l $PaCO_2$ <4.5kPa). Results from hyperventilation. Causes can include panic attacks and sepsis. Symptoms may consist of light-headedness, numbness, tingling, confusion, inability to concentrate, dry mouth, diaphoresis.

**Metabolic acidosis** (pH <7.35 mmol/l bicarbonate ($HCO_3$) <22 mmol/l).

Failure to remove/buffer sufficient H+ which is caused by excessive production or accumulation of renal acids (renal failure); lactic acids (circulatory failure); ketoacids (diabetic ketoacidosis); ingestion of acids, e.g. salicylates and loss of base (associated with diarrhoea, causing metabolic acidosis). Symptoms include headache, confusion, lethargy, reduced levels of consciousness, cardiac arrhythmias, kussmaul respiration (deep, rapid breathing). Acidosis causes hyperventilation (body's attempting to 'blow off' $CO_2$ and compensate for acidosis).

**Metabolic alkalosis** (pH >7.45 mmol/l $HCO_3$ >26 mmol/l). Caused by a loss of acids (excessive vomiting/gastric drainage; potassium depletion through diuretic therapy; burns and by excess of base acids (from ingestion of acids/excessive use of bicarbonate). Symptoms include dizziness, muscle twitching/cramps, nausea/vomiting, respiratory depression.

**FIGURE 4.8** Interpreting arterial blood gas (ABG) 1

# INTERPRETING ARTERIAL BLOOD GAS (ABG) 2

**Bicarbonate (HCO3) (Normal 22–26mmol/l)**
The main chemical buffer in plasma, mainly produced in the liver and kidneys. It provides information regarding how much alkali is in the blood. HCo3 also indicates how well the metabolic system is functioning (linking closely to kidney function – excretion).
To maintain pH within normal range, the kidneys excrete or retain HCO3. In the event of acidosis HCO3, is retained (levels increased). With alkalosis, excretion of HCO3 (levels reduced).

**Base excess (normal -2 to +2mmol/l)**
This represents the amount of excess/insufficient level of bicarbonate in the system i.e. amount of acid or base required to store one litre of blood to its normal pH. Only the metabolic component is reflected. In the case of metabolic acidosis, acid needs to be added to return pH to normal, therefore base excess is negative. For metabolic alkalosis, acid needs to be removed, hence base excess is positive. Zero is a neutral score.

**Oxygen (PaO2) (normal 11.5–13.5 kPa)**
PaO2 is not directly associated or influences acid base balance. It provides information about respiratory function. PaO2 is the measurement of partial pressure of oxygen dissolved in arterial blood and is dependent upon the effectiveness of gas exchange. It is vital for the survival of cells.

**Carbon dioxide (PaCO2) (normal 4.5–6.0 kPa)**
CO2 is a cellular waste product of metabolism and is transported to the lungs in plasma in the form of carbonic acid (H2CO3). It provides information concerning ventilation. PaCO2 is used as a guide to measure CO2 in the blood and referred to as the respiratory parameter.

Note that those with chronic obstructive disorders develop alterations in gas exchange as a result of adjusting and becoming use to a high PaCO2. The central chemoreceptors become tolerant to high CO2 levels. If given too much oxygen (O2), this drive will be inhibited causing respiratory failure. The respiratory stimulant becomes hypoxia (known as the hypoxic drive). Low PaCO2 levels will eventually inhibit respiratory stimulation, resulting in an initial increase in the respiratory rate but eventually becoming slower and more shallow (leading to type 11 respiratory failure). Hypercapnia (PaCO2 greater than 6.0 kPa (BTS, 2017) stimulates the respiratory centre to increase the rate and depth of breathing.

**Compensation** – The aim is homeostasis (normal acid base balance). Buffers, carbonic acid and bicarbonate are combined in 1:20 ratio) i.e. 1 carbonic acid to 20 bicarbonate molecules. In order to maintain the 1:20 ratio, when carbonic acid levels increase, so do bicarbonate levels and when carbonic acid levels decrease, so do bicarbonate levels. If the pH becomes abnormal, the body will attempt to return it to normal through compensation. In compensation, the system NOT experiencing problems (i.e. respiratory or renal) will attempt to correct the 1:20 ratio, to return the pH to normal.

Therefore one system compensates for the other. So, blood values will not be as we expect them to be, i.e. movement in the opposite direction. For example, respiratory disturbances are compensated by the renal system and metabolic disturbances by the respiratory system. Respiratory compensatory response is not fully activated until 24 -48 hours after initial activation. Respiratory compensation occurs at a faster rate than renal. Any acute respiratory problem will always be uncompensated as the kidneys will not have time to compensate.

**Interpreting ABG**
Questions to ask...

- Look at the pH – is there acidaemia or alkalaemia?
- Look at the PaCO2 – is it high, low or normal?
- Look at the PaO2 – is the patient hypoxaemic?
- Look at the HCO3 – is it high, low or normal?
- Is compensation occurring?

**FIGURE 4.9** Interpreting arterial blood gas (ABG) 2

# INTRAPLEURAL CHEST DRAIN

Chest drains remove any abnormal collection of fluid, blood, pus or air from thorax. Chest drains are used to treat pneumothorax and pleural effusions.

Pneumothorax symptoms

- Tachypnoea
- Respiratory distress and/or arrest
- Unilaterally decreased or absent lung sounds
- Tachycardia
- Mental status changes, including decreased alertness and/or consciousness
- Low oxygen saturation levels
- Cyanosis
- Jugular venous distension (with a tension pneumothorax)
- Hypotension (key sign of a tension pneumothorax)

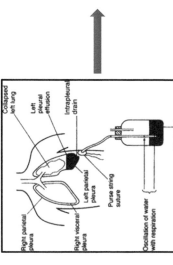

Complications

➢ Tension pneumothorax – life threatening. Increasing trapped air within the pleural space. Mediastinal structures shifted to the opposite side with cardiopulmonary function compromised.

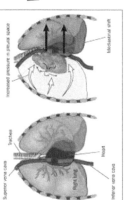

Tension Pneumothorax

**FIGURE 4.10** Intrapleural chest drain

# CARE OF CHEST DRAIN

**Care of the chest drain**

- ONLY clamp drain if disconnected (risk of tension pneumothorax).
- Never lift bottle above chest level.
- Negative pressure suction may be used. Stop immediately if pain or shortness of breath is present.
- Conduct a full respiratory assessment and monitor frequently. Monitor for signs of infection (wound and chest).
- Monitoring of amount and character of drainage.
- Ensure no kinks in tubing and connections are secure.
- Note any air leakage (bubbles in drainage system). Lung may not be re-expanded.
- If blocked 'milk' the tubes with a roller clamp.
- Daily dressing change.

Chest drain should not be left in situ >3 weeks due to risk of:

- ascending infection
- erosion intercostal vessels
- haemorrhage
- local inflammation, adhesion

Remove when there are no air leaks for 24 hours; drainage is <100ml/day; complete lung re-expansion.

**Changing of drain bottle**

1. Wash hands.
2. Use personal protective equipment.
3. Aseptic technique, remove the new unit from packaging and place adjacent to old drain.
4. Follow manufacturer's guidance to prepare the chest drain.
5. Clamp drainage tube (prevent air entering chest).
6. Disconnect old bottle as per manufacturer's guidance.
7. Insert the tubing into the new bottle; you may hear it click.
8. Unclamp the drainage tube.
9. If on drainage, resume.
10. Place old chamber into appropriate waste bag.
11. Wash hands and document.

**Removal of chest drain (NOT by student nurses)**

- DO NOT clamp the chest drain. Chest drain should be oscillating (swinging). Chest X-ray before procedure.
- Remove dressing and cut suture.
- Place a gauze pad and dressing over the chest tube exit site.
- Tell the patient to take a deep breath and perform the Valsalva manoeuvre (this will forcibly inflate the lung against chest wall = positive pressure in pleural space). Pull out tube while covering exit site.
- Patient should hold their breath until purse-string suture is tied. Apply a fresh dressing.
- CXR after 24 hours and before discharge.

**FIGURE 4.11** Care of chest drain

## Activity: now test yourself

1. What are the signs of respiratory failure?

   a) bradypnoea, bradycardia, confusion, cyanosis

   b) tachypnoea, tachycardia, confusion, cyanosis

   c) tachypnoea, tachycardia, orientated, no cyanosis

   d) normal respiratory rate, tachycardia, orientated, cyanosis.

2. List three indications for the insertion of a tracheostomy tube.

3. True or false? The changing of a tracheostomy dressing is a two-person procedure.

4. What is the difference between a fenestrated and non-fenestrated tracheostomy tube?

5. What type of tracheostomy tube should a speaking valve be used with?

**Answers**

1. b) tachypnoea, tachycardia, confusion, cyanosis.

2. Any of the following: to reduce the work of breathing, insertion of an endotracheal tube, bypass severe acute upper airway obstruction, remove excessive bronchial secretions.

3. True. *One person should hold the tube in place while the other person performs the dressing.*

4. Fenestrated tubes have single or multiple holes; non-fenestrated tubes do not have any holes.

5. Uncuffed and fenestrated tube (with fenestrated inner cannula).

## Reflection: ask yourself

1. What do I know now that I didn't know before?

2. What am I confused/unclear about?

3. What areas do I need to focus on?

4. My action plan for further learning (make objectives SMART – Specific/Measurable/Achievable/Realistic/Time-bound):

# CHAPTER 5

# Cardiovascular skills

Tina Moore

## Overview

The cardiovascular system plays a pivotal role in sustaining life alongside the respiratory system. It has a responsibility to deliver oxygenated blood, nutrients and other substances to cells and to remove waste products such as carbon dioxide. The cardiovascular system also plays a key role in thermoregulation and blood clotting.

The heart pumps deoxygenated blood to the tissues and cells. Through homeostasis it controls blood pressure.

The vascular system delivers oxygen, nutrients and other substances to the cells and removes the waste products of cellular metabolism. The vascular system is made up of arteries, arterioles, capillaries, venules and veins.

## Link to *Future Nurse Proficiencies* (NMC 2018)

*Platform 3* Assessing needs and planning care (Sections 3.2; 3.4; 3.5).

**Annexe B, Part 1**: Procedures for assessing people's needs for person-centred care. Specifically, 2.3: set up and manage routine electrocardiogram (ECG) investigations and interpret normal and commonly encountered abnormal traces and 2.5: manage and interpret cardiac monitors, infusion pumps, blood glucose monitors and other monitoring devices.

**Annexe B, Part 2**: Procedures for the planning, provision and management of person-centred nursing care. Specifically, 3.5: take appropriate action to reduce or minimise pain or discomfort.

## Expected knowledge

- Anatomy and physiology of the cardiovascular system
- Physiology of the conduction pathway
- Chapter 1, Anatomy and physiology of the cardiovascular system.

## Introduction

Cardiovascular function is often compromised in patients who become acutely unwell; therefore assessing and monitoring cardiovascular function is critical when caring for such patients. Whilst extremely important, there are limitations to basic monitoring (e.g. of pulse, blood pressure) as they only provide some of the haemodynamic information required.

Often, when the patient's compensatory mechanisms are no longer enough to sustain normal physiological functioning, the patient will deteriorate and become acutely/critically ill. In these instances there is a need to use more complex approaches to assessment and care management, making it necessary to use more complex devices and equipment.

## Content

| Related physiology | Procedure for measuring central venous pressure (CVP) | Assessment of pulse deficit |
|---|---|---|
| Recognition of common arrhythmias | Formulae for measuring the mean arterial pressure (MAP) | Procedure for measuring capillary refill time (CRT) |

## Learning outcomes

- Understand the rationale for and significance of haemodynamic assessment
- Demonstrate the correct techniques for measuring CVP, MAP, CRT
- Recognise common arrhythmias
- Identify the main causes of high and low CVP measurements.

## Key background

The presence of such assessment and monitoring devices should not detract from the fact that fundamental nursing assessment should still be performed. For example the manual taking of a pulse: if the patient is attached to a cardiac monitor, the monitor will only display the rate and rhythm (unless the patient has an arterial then pulse pressures can be monitored). In a general ward area, electronic pulse pressures are not normally monitored. Therefore, without taking a manual pulse vital information about pulse volume will be lost. Pulse volume can provide information about the patient's circulatory status, e.g. a 'weak and thready' pulse normally indicates low cardiac output possibly due to fluid deficit, or a 'strong and bounding' one is possibly due to fluid overload.

Apex and radial assessment should be performed in order to determine the pulse deficit. Assessing the radial pulse alone will not provide a true picture of the patient's heart rate. The apex and radial assessment is required when the patient has an irregular pulse (such as in atrial fibrillation or atrial flutter). The pulse deficit is the difference between the heart rate and the pulse rate and determines that ventricular contraction may not be sufficiently strong enough to transmit an arterial pulse wave through the peripheral artery.

Today, mean arterial pressure (MAP) measurements are being relied upon more as a marker for cardiovascular deterioration or improvement, particularly with acutely/critically ill patients, as MAP provides an average blood pressure across the cardiac cycle and offers a better indication than either systolic or diastolic pressures as to whether the patient's brain and other vital organs are receiving sufficient oxygen. These measurements are used to evaluate the perfusion of vital body organs and are used for the goal and evaluation criteria in the physiological responses to interventions thus increasing blood pressure.

The cardiac output (flow), systemic vascular resistance (pressure) and central venous pressure (resistance) determine the MAP. So, MAP = (CO x SVR) + CVP. These measurements provide more in-depth knowledge relating to the patient's cardiovascular status, giving information about approximate perfusion pressures at organ and cellular levels.

The average MAP is 70100 mmHg. A MAP below 65 mmHg results in hypotension, poor perfusion, poor oxygenation to vital

69

organs and peripheries; below 60 mmHg is considered incompatible with life. A high reading of above 110 mmHg indicates hypertension.

Automated blood pressure machines and most monitors at the bedside will automatically calculate the MAP. Where such devices are not available, the MAP should be calculated manually. It is good practice to calculate the MAP manually when using an automated device at least once per shift and of course when there are discrepancies between the patient's condition, blood pressure readings and automated MAP readings.

Capillary refill time (CRT) is the time taken for the colour to return to an external capillary bed after the application of pressure causing blanching. CRT is a non-invasive, quick and straightforward assessment. Whilst a simple technique, it is a very important one as it can provide quick information regarding the patient's cardiovascular and perfusion status. CRT is considered a 'red flag' procedure, helping to identify those who are acutely/critically ill, particularly in the case of children.

Whilst blood pressure measurements, mean arterial pressure and capillary refill time provide some essential information they do not provide information about intravascular blood volume, vascular tone, effectiveness of right ventricular function, pulmonary vascular resistance or intrathoracic pressure.

Central venous pressure (CVP) measurements are often used to provide more in-depth knowledge of the patient's cardiovascular status. CVP is the measurement of the blood pressure in the right atrium of the heart. Although the CVP does not measure blood volume directly, it can provide some information about intravascular volume, venous return, venous tone and intrathoracic pressure. The use of CVP monitoring can provide early recognition of fluid imbalances and cardiac dysfunction. Remember, this is crucial for acutely/critically ill patients. Indications for central venous access would be for those patients who for example are in shock and require haemodynamic monitoring and rapid administration of intravenous fluids. The most common routes used are the internal jugular vein, subclavian vein and femoral vein (which has a higher risk of infection and haemorrhage).

Irregularities of the rhythm necessitate an ECG (12 lead) assessment and sometimes continuous ECG monitoring for arrhythmias. ECGs are the most commonly conducted cardiovascular diagnostic procedure used to diagnose or exclude cardiac arrhythmias and indeed cardiac disease. Whilst the ECG is used for diagnostic purposes, nurses should nevertheless be able to recognise common arrhythmias. Monitoring without the staff being able to interpret the monitoring induces a dangerous false sense of security.

Cardiac monitoring is a useful and non-invasive method of monitoring the patient's cardiac status. There are a number of arrhythmia specialist nurses who specifically work with and contribute to the care of patients with arrhythmias. This is a relatively new role.

# APEX AND RADIAL ASSESSMENT

This assessment is required for a cardiac condition known as atrial fibrillation (full explanation on page 74) or when the patients pulse rhythm is irregular. The irregularity is caused by a difference between the heart rate and the pulse. This is known as the 'pulse deficit'.

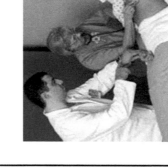

**The procedure for assessing apex and radial**

1. Wash and dry hands before and after procedure.
2. Explain the procedure and its purpose (this will help reduce any anxieties that will influence the heart rate) and where possible, gain consent.
3. This procedure requires two people – one to assess the apical pulse and the other to assess the radial pulse. This assessment also requires effective coordination.
4. The apical pulse is listened to through a stethoscope.
5. Locate the pulse site on the left side of the chest (apex of the heart). Put the diaphragm of the stethoscope over the apical pulse and listen for heart sounds, which sound like 'lub dub'.
6. At the same time, the second person should locate the radial pulse.
7. A watch with a second had should be visible to both people undertaking the assessment.
8. At the same time both the apex pulse and radial pulse are counted for one full minute. Hence, starting and finishing times should be the same.
9. One person should take responsibility to indicate when to start counting and when to finish. Apart from the rate, rhythm and depth (radial pulse volume) should also be noted.

**Top tip:**
Ensure that the apex rate, the radial pulse rate and the difference between the two (pulse deficit) are recorded and documented. In health, the pulse deficit should be zero. A pulse deficit occurs when some of the chaotic impulses from the sinoatrial node do not filter through the atrioventricular node and the rest of the conducting system.

In the instance of a patient with atrial fibrillation the recording could be as follows:

Apex pulse rate is 124, radial pulse rate 96, making the pulse deficit = 28 bpm.

The apex pulse will ALWAYS be higher or equal to the radial pulse, never lower.

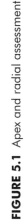

**FIGURE 5.1** Apex and radial assessment

# ARRHYTHMIA RECOGNITION 1

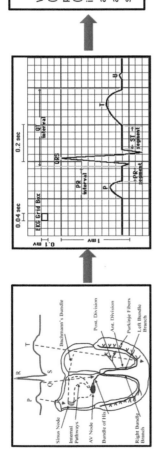

Conducting pathway

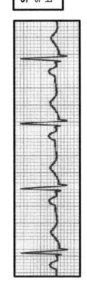

ECG trace on paper

When assessing ECG always note blood pressure (signs of shock), chest pain (cardiac ischaemia), pulmonary oedema (heart failure), syncope (reduced blood flow to the brain). Other influencing factors affecting the heart rhythm are blood potassium (K +), magnesium (Mg++) and calcium Ca++), therefore blood levels should be checked and monitored closely.

**Sinus rhythm** P wave followed by QRS complex; P-R interval regular normal (0.12 – 0.20 seconds); QRS complex normal (less than 0.12 seconds; R-R interval regular Rate 60 – 100 beats per minute).

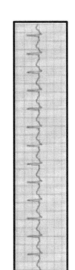

**Sinus tachycardia** (Not viewed as an arrhythmia). P wave followed by QRS complex; R-R interval regular; Rate (at rest) >than 100 bpm.

**FIGURE 5.2** Arrhythmia recognition 1

# ARRHYTHMIA RECOGNITION 2

## Atrial fibrillation

A large number of disorganised electrical impulses sent from the Sino Atrial node. Some will transmit to the Atrio Ventricular node, then follow the normal conducting pathway. Apex beat is greater than radial beat. P wave is absent; normal QRS complex; R-R interval irregular; Rate (ventricular/pulse) 110–200 bpm (atrial rate >300 bpm).

Identify pulse deficit through apex and radial assessment.

## Atrial flutter

The SA node sends a premature electrical signal that moves in an organized circular motion, or 'circuit', causing the atria only to contract. The second impulse will follow the normal conducting pathway (known as 2:1 block).

P wave is replaced with 'saw tooth' pattern; normal QRS complex and T wave; R-R interval irregular regular (usually 2:1 block); Rate (ventricular/pulse) 125 – 150 bpm (atrial rate >300 bpm).

## Supra-ventricular tachycardia (SVT)

Rapid abnormal heart rhythm. P wave is not easily identifiable; QRS complex is narrow; R-R interval irregular when premature beat occurs; Rate >140 bpm.

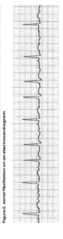
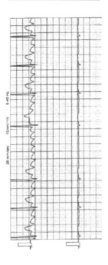
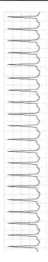

**FIGURE 5.3** Arrhythmia recognition 2

# ARRHYTHMIA RECOGNITION 3

## Premature Ventricular Contraction (PVC)

The ventricle initiates these premature beats. Complexes look very wide and unusual. Absent P wave absent; QRS complex looks wide (> 0.1 second); T wave absent; R-R interval irregular when premature beat occurs.

- ➤ Note: *Count* how many per minute. The more per minute – the more dangerous the arrhythmia is (initiating ventricular tachycardia (VT)).
- ➤ *Pattern* (i.e. occurring every second beat (bigeminy) or third beat (trigeminy)).
- ➤ *Shape* (indicates location of beat).
- ➤ *Position* to previous complex (particularly T wave). An ectopic beat occurring repolarisation (T wave) is known as 'R on T' phenomenon and can deteriorate to VT very quickly.

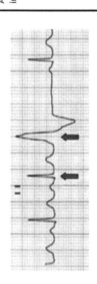

## Ventricular tachycardia (VT)

Impulses are activated by the ventricles only. P wave usually buried in QRS complex; QRS complex looks wide and unusual; R-R interval usually regular; Ventricular rate is 150–250 bpm. Cardiac output may be maintained – no loss of consciousness. BUT THIS WILL NOT LAST FOR LONG PERIODS OF TIME. An emergency/cardiac arrest situation.

## Ventricular fibrillation (VF)

VF is a rapid, uncoordinated quivering contractions of the ventricles. Ventricular rate is 150–250 bpm. There is no audible heartbeat or palpable pulse. Cardiac arrest situation.

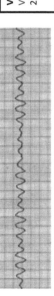

**FIGURE 5.4** Arrhythmia recognition 3

# ARRHYTHMIA RECOGNITION 4

## Bradycardia

A slow heartbeat of <60 bpm). Causes include hypothermia, hypothyroidism, beta blockers/digoxin, ischemia, and hypoxaemia. It may also be a natural physiological response – i.e. in athletes.

P wave and QRS complex present. R-R interval regular; Rate is <60 bpm.

## Conduction abnormalities

### First degree AV block

P wave present but P-R interval is prolonged (>0.2 seconds); normal QRS complex; R-R interval regular; Rate is 60–100 bpm.

### Second degree AV block (Mobitz type 1/Wenckebach)

P wave present but P-R interval is progressively prolonged (until P wave is not conducted (i.e. until a drop beat is seen)); P-R interval is not constant; normal QRS complex; rate is 60–80 bpm; R-R interval shortens as the P-R interval prolongs; after each dropped beat the P-R interval is normal and the cycle starts again.

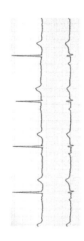

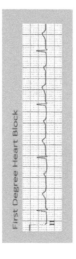
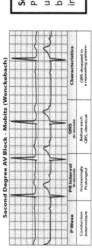

**FIGURE 5.5** Arrhythmia recognition 4

# ARRHYTHMIA RECOGNITION 5

**Second degree AV block (2:1)**
Ratio of two P waves to one QRS; Constant P-R interval; normal QRS complex; rate is 60–80 bpm; R-R interval is regular.

**Third degree AV block (complete heart block)**
Complete block of the atrial impulses occurs at the A-V junction. Another pacemaker distal to the block takes over in order to activate the ventricles. Causes include digitalis toxicity, acute infection, myocardial infarction.
Complete dissociation between P waves and QRS complex; P-R interval is not constant; a greater number of P waves that QRS complex; atrial rate is normal but ventricular rate is slow, <40; R-R interval is relatively constant.

**Asystole**
Absent P, QRS, T waves; no rate; no palpable pulse or breathing.
This is a cardiac arrest situation.

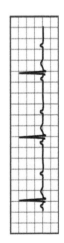

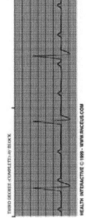

THIRD DEGREE <COMPLETE> AV BLOCK

HEALTH INTERACTIVE © 1999 - WWW.RNCEUS.COM

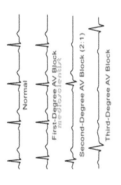

Normal

First-Degree AV Block

Second-Degree AV Block (2:1)

Third-Degree AV Block

Comparison of the heart blocks

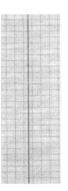

**FIGURE 5.6** Arrhythmia recognition 5

# CENTRAL VENOUS PRESSURE MEASUREMENT (CVP)

CVP monitoring provides information about intravascular volume, venous return, venous tone and intrathoracic pressure. It can provide early recognition of fluid imbalances and cardiac dysfunction.

All observations of the patient (i.e. clinical signs, vital signs) need to be considered when interpreting results.

Uses for CVP monitoring:

➤ Continuous haemodynamic monitoring (shock).
➤ Rapid administration of intravenous fluids.
➤ Secure venous access for the infusion of drugs that cause irritation of the veins or that is administered directly into the heart (inotropic drugs).
➤ Evaluation response to fluid resuscitation/inotropic support.
➤ Frequent blood sampling (particularly in children).
➤ Venous access that cannot be obtained by other venous routes (e.g. femoral vein).

## Insertion sites

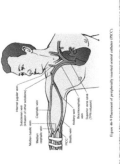

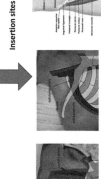

Internal Jugular          Subclavian          Femoral

## Peripherally inserted central catheter (PICC)

The basilic, cephalic or brachial veins may be used. PICC can also be used for a range of treatments such as chemotherapy, blood transfusion, antibiotic therapy, IV therapy and withdrawal of blood. The line is a long, thin, flexible catheter that has a longer life shelf than those used for CVP.

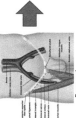

Figure 46-9 Placement of peripherally inserted central catheter (PICC)

## Complications

*Haemorrhage* from catheter site or disconnection of line. Patients with coagulation disorders are at risk.

*Occlusion* of the catheter from a thrombus or kinked tube. Keep line patent by a slow infusion. The risk is increased if the patient is mobile. Positioning of the unconscious patient may cause accidental occlusion or dislodgment.

*Infection* – note any redness, pain, swelling around the catheter site. Send swabs for culture and sensitivity (C & S) if indicated. Strict asepsis is critical.

*Air embolus* – lines that become disconnected should be checked before measuring CVP.

*Catheter displacement* – can cause arrhythmias and should be reported immediately.

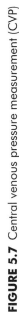

**FIGURE 5.7** Central venous pressure measurement (CVP)

# MEASURING A CVP

## Procedure

- Explain procedure and gain consent if possible. Wash and dry hands before and after procedure.
- Check patency of the line (flush with 3–5mls of fluid). Initially the white arrow (on the three way tap) is turned straight up towards the manometer (fluid flow from fluid bag to the patient's Central Venous Catheter (CVC). If fluid does not flow freely the line has to be 'unblocked' before proceeding. Any fluid from infused into the patient should be recorded on the fluid balance chart (crucial in patients with fluid balance problems and children).
- If possible use supine position. If not, then use the semi recumbent position. Ensure consistency and use the same position for measurements. Document position used.
- Position manometer at level of right atrium. Use mid axilla point (phlebostaticaxis) for measurements. Place the manometer arm at the level of right atrium. Place an 'x' on the patient's skin to mark the position.
- Zero the manometer by moving the manometer scale up or down to allow the bubble to be aligned with zero.

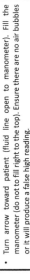

- Turn arrow toward patient (fluid line open to manometer). Fill the manometer (do not to fill right to the top). Ensure there are no air bubbles or it will produce a false high reading.
- If air is present in the manometer or fluid line (going to the manometer), turn the clamps on (luer lock connection otherwise blood will flow out of the CVC). Disconnect the IV line and let the fluids run until all air is purged from the system. Reopen the luer lock connection. Requires strict asepsis.
- Turn arrow toward the fluid line closing this and opening the connection between the patient and manometer.
- Observe the falling level in the manometer, fluid will run into the patient's CVC until the height of the fluid column exerts a pressure equivalent to the patient's central venous pressure.
- The top of the fluid column will slightly oscillate as the patient breathes. Record mean level (where the fluid in the spirit level hovers).
- Reposition and make patient comfortable.
- Generally, 'normal' values are considered to be 5–10 cmH2o (manual) and 2-6 mmHg (monitor) for both adult and child.

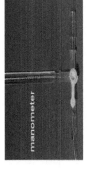

## Causes of increased CVP

- Hypervolaemia, heart failure
- Cardiac incompetence
- Increased intrathoracic pressure (tension pneumothorax, pulmonary embolism)
- Obstructed or displaced catheter tip; incorrect measuring technique
(**Clinical signs**: tachypnoea, dyspnoea, shallow breath and signs of pulmonary oedema)

## Causes of decreased CVP

- Increased vasodilation (vasogenic shock)
- Hypovolaemia, dehydration
- Incorrect measuring technique
(**Clinical signs**: hypotension, tachycardia, oliguria)

**FIGURE 5.8** Measuring a CVP

# MEAN ARTERIAL PRESSURE (MAP) AND CAPILLIARY REFILL TIME (CRT)

## Mean Arterial Pressure (MAP)

MAP is used to evaluate the perfusion of vital body organs the physiological responses to interventions increasing blood pressure. The MAP measures the average blood pressure over the entire cardiac cycle of systole and diastole. Measurements provide more in-depth knowledge relating to the patient's cardiovascular status, giving information about approximate perfusion pressures at organ and cellular levels.

## Measuring MAP

MAP is determined by the cardiac output (CO) (*flow*), systemic vascular resistance (SVR) (*pressure*) and central venous pressure (CVP) (*resistance*). MAP = (CO x SVR) + CVP.

The equation for manual calculation of the MAP is systolic + (diastolic x 2) ÷ 3.

For example – a B/P of 120 (systolic) / 90 (diastolic) = MAP 100 mmHg

> ➤ 120 + (90 x 2 = 180) = 120 + 180 = 300. 300 divided by 3 = 100
> ➤ B/P of 66 (systolic) / 40 (diastolic) = 49 mmHg (rounded up)
> ➤ 66 + (40 x 2 = 80) = 66 + 146. 146 divided by 3 = 48.66 (49 rounded up)

Below 60 mmHg – incompatible with life

Average MAP – 70–100 mmHg

Above 110 mmHg – hypertension

---

Capillary refill time (CRT) is defined as the time taken for colour to return to an external capillary bed after pressure is applied to cause blanching. It is a quick, easy and non-invasive procedure. CRT is dependent on the visual inspection of blood returning to the distal capillaries after they have been emptied by the application of external pressure.

CRT is a simple and quick test requiring minimal equipment or time to perform. The finger is the preferred site but the sternum and forehead can also be used. Avoid performing this procedure in environments with poor lighting and a patient who is cold or peripherally shut down.

## Procedure for taking CRT

1. Wash hands before and after the procedure.
2. Explain procedure (and potential discomfort). Where possible, gain consent.
3. Ideally, position limb at approximately the same level as the heart. Remove any nail polish.
4. Press firmly on the patient's nailbed with your thumb for five seconds (blanching the skin).
5. Release the pressure (checking to see that the skin was blanched). Note the time that it takes for the area to return to normal colour, or the same colour as the surrounding skin (CRT).
6. Record your findings/escalate if indicated.

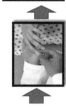

Normal CRT is <2 seconds or less. Anything above this (i.e. 3 or greater) is abnormal, particularly for babies (over 7 days), infants, toddlers and children.

A slow CRT may indicate dehydration/shock/hypothermia/peripheral vascular disease.

**FIGURE 5.9** Mean arterial pressure (MAP) and capillary refill time (CRT)

**Activity: now test yourself**

1. What is the purpose of an apex and radial assessment?

2. Which of the following is not considered an arrhythmia?

   a)  ventricular tachycardia

   b)  sinus tachycardia

   c)  atrial fibrillation

   d)  sinus rhythm.

3. List four reasons for CVP monitoring.

4. What is the difference between MAP and CRT?

5. Which of the following statements is false?

   a)  CRT assessment is quick and simple.

   b)  The normal CRT is less than two seconds.

   c)  It is best to count the seconds out loud.

   d)  A slow CRT may indicate low blood volume, shock, dehydration.

## Answers

1. Apex and radial assessment is used to determine how many ventricular contractions are not sufficiently strong enough to transmit an arterial pulse wave through the peripheral artery. The pulse deficit is the difference between the heart rate and the pulse rate.

2. d) sinus rhythm is not considered to be an arrhythmia.

3. Reasons for CVP monitoring include:

   a) *continuous haemodynamic monitoring*

   b) *rapid administration of fluids intravenously*

   c) *the infusion of highly irritant drugs*

   d) *to evaluate fluid resuscitation or inotropic support*

   e) *frequent blood sampling*

   f) *venous access (patient peripherally shut down).*

4. MAP is used to evaluate the perfusion of vital body organs and to measure the physiological responses to interventions to increase blood pressure. There is a formula to measure the MAP.

   CRT measures peripheral perfusion. This is done by pressing on the finger digit for five seconds.

5. c) It is best to count the seconds out loud.

   *It is more accurate to measure using a timer such as a watch or clock with a second hand rather than counting out loud.*

**Reflection: ask yourself**

1. What do I know now that I didn't know before?

2. What am I confused/unclear about?

3. What areas do I need to focus on?

4. My action plan for learning (make objectives SMART – Specific/Measurable/Achievable/Realistic/Time-bound):

# CHAPTER 6

# Cannulation and venepuncture

*Sheila Cunningham*

## Overview

The NMC (2018) in their recently produced standards of nurse proficiency extended the range of skills and tasks that qualifying nurses ought to be able to perform. Two of these were previously the domain of medical or other staff: venepuncture and cannulation. These skills are not new to nurses. Many practitioners and nurses working in specialist areas have been undertaking them for many years. However it is now something expected of all nurses and so must be viewed as part of nursing care and practiced with dexterity as well as compassion and care.

### Link to *Future Nurse Proficiencies* (NMC 2018)

**Annexe B**: Nursing procedures Section 2: Procedures for assessing people's needs for person-centred care. Specifically, 2.2: undertake venepuncture and cannulation and blood sampling, interpreting normal and common abnormal blood profiles and venous blood gases.

### Expected knowledge

- The rationale for taking blood tests and the ranges of normal for key parameters (gases and electrolytes)
- Health and safety procedures for dealing with and discarding blood and sharps.

## Introduction

Blood tests are one of the most commonly used diagnostic aids in the care and evaluation of patients. They can offer valuable information on a person's nutritional, metabolic, biochemical and haematological status. The skill of taking or drawing blood requires a great deal of practice and knowledge prior to engaging with real-life patients. It is invasive and can hurt, whether or not individuals have a fear of needles. Many areas have trained professionals called phlebotomists whose role is to take blood; however, this skill is increasingly expected of all nurses within the UK. Nurses are in an ideal position to take blood from patients as it allows for a more patient-centred approach, especially with anxious patients or children. Nurses are central to care and thus can gauge a patient's reaction and use their rapport to enable this painful but essential task to be completed. As always, nurses ought to work within their sphere of competence and this entails knowing not just the technique but also the relevant anatomy of veins to proceed competently.

## Content

| Selecting veins | Order of blood sampling | Venepuncture procedure |
|---|---|---|
| Cannulation procedure | Complications of cannulation | Rationale for venepuncture an cannulation |

## Learning outcomes

- Discuss the purpose of venepuncture and cannulation
- Analyse the preparations and complications which may occur in these invasive procedures
- Explain the principles and procedures of cannulation and potential complications of siting cannula inappropriately
- Explain the principles and procedures of venepuncture and the safety precautions around this.

## Key background

Increasing numbers of patients are having vascular access devices (VADs) inserted either short- or long-term and thus healthcare professionals ought to be prepared with the appropriate knowledge and skills to optimise care. The aim of intravenous access management is the safe and effective delivery of treatment without discomfort or tissue damage and without compromising venous access. This is especially important if long-term therapy is proposed (Lister, Hofland and Grafton, 2020). Due to issues such as the delegation of cannulating to junior or poorly prepared staff, the frequency with which the skill is performed and the serious nature of complications and ensuing poor experience by patients (Moreau et al., 2012), the UK Infection Prevention Society (IPS) has produced a vessel health and preservation (VHP) framework (Hallam et al., 2016) to address these issues with a comprehensive decision-making tool. It originated in the United States but is now adapted for use in the United Kingdom and addresses key concerns for intravenous access, the duration and type of medication but also patient lifestyle in the choice of device and vein integrity. It refers to cannulation, but is useful in addressing decision-making for all such invasive procedures.

Phlebotomy is the practice of taking or drawing blood. It has been practised for centuries and is still a common invasive procedure in health care. There are three methods of obtaining blood specimens: skin puncture (for example blood sugar finger stab), venepuncture and arterial puncture. Each step in the process of phlebotomy affects the quality of the specimen, a fundamental issue in preventing laboratory error, patient injury or discomfort or even death. For example, touching the arms or location to verify the location of a vein before insertion of the needle increases the chance that a specimen will be contaminated. All these procedures are invasive and require aseptic techniques. Despite the evidence highlighting that patients often find venepuncture distressing and painful, very little literature exists relating to interventions aiming to reduce fear, pain and anxiety (RCN 2016a). Furthermore, they are potentially anxiety-provoking and so a calm and confident demeanour can help. Children and young people may be particularly anxious and fearful of needles and so knowledge and use of preparatory creams or gels to 'numb' the area prior to venepuncture or cannulation may be useful. There are considerable physical, emotional and comprehension differences between children of varying ages, and it is recommended that practitioners develop competence within specific age bands according to their area of practice (RCN, 2016b).

Since venepuncture and cannulation are invasive skills there are also serious professional and legal considerations. Nurses are responsible and accountable for the care they give which includes these skills. This includes not only actions but omissions which therefore emphasises the need to be fully prepared and confident in the skills and procedures. Nurses owe their patients a duty of care to ensure their safety and wellbeing. Breaching that duty of care makes them liable. Such breaches could include not carrying out tasks to the required standard. A further key responsibility is documentation of interventions. In terms of cannulation, recordkeeping is essential and a critical responsibility of nurses. Documentation ought to clearly identify site selection, number of attempts and any problems encountered during the procedure. The record should be signed and dated with the time of insertion. Furthermore, records should demonstrate the care of the peripheral device as well as the outcome of treatment (Lister, Hofland and Grafton, 2020). One further consideration is consent by the patient to the procedure and treatment. Throughout this series of skill books this aspect is emphasised.

# VENEPUNCTURE AND CANNULATION – WHAT IS IT?

## Venepuncture

Describes the procedure of inserting a needle into a vein, usually for the purpose of withdrawing blood for haematological, biochemical or bacteriological analysis.

- One of the most commonly performed procedures within healthcare situations.
- Ought not cause discomfort.
- Requires a good understanding of the arteries, veins and associated nerves within the arm.

Also referred to as: *vascular access device (VAD)*.

## Legal and professional issues

*Accountability*
- Promote and safeguard the interests of patients (act or omission).
- Maintain and improve professional knowledge.
- Evidence based practice

*Duty of care:*
- Work within sphere of competency (i.e. adequate training).
- Acknowledge own limitations.

*Liability:*
- Authorised to perform the task.
- If harm/injury caused.

*Record keeping:*
- Of: site selection, number of attempts and any problems encountered during the procedure.
- Dated and signed.

*Consent*
- Informed and voluntary.

## Cannulation

- *Intravenous (IV) cannulation* is a technique in which a cannula is placed inside a vein to provide access.
- This VAD allows for samples of blood to be taken as well as the administration of fluids, medications, nutrition, chemotherapy, and blood products.

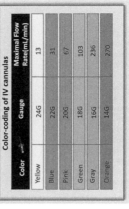

Figure 1 Venflon device for cannulation (BD/Becton Dickinson Infusion Therapy AB)

| Color-coding of IV cannulas | | |
|---|---|---|
| Color | Gauge | Maximal Flow Rate(mL/min) |
| Yellow | 24G | 13 |
| Blue | 22G | 31 |
| Pink | 20G | 67 |
| Green | 18G | 103 |
| Gray | 16G | 236 |
| Orange | 14G | 270 |

Figure 2 Colour of cannulae and associated lumen size and fluid flow rate.

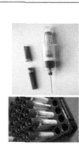

Figure 3 Blood collection tubes (Creative Commons Public Domain)

## Considerations

For successful venepuncture and cannulation
- The choice of vein and location.
- Choice of venepuncture device.
- Asepsis.
- Safe technique and practices.

**FIGURE 6.1** Venepuncture and cannulation: what is it?

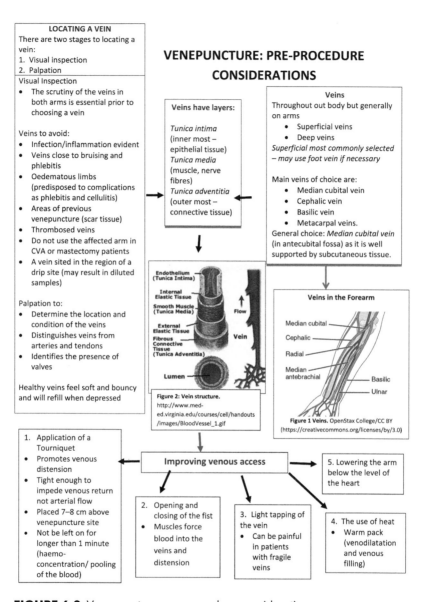

**LOCATING A VEIN**
There are two stages to locating a vein:
1. Visual inspection
2. Palpation

**Visual Inspection**
- The scrutiny of the veins in both arms is essential prior to choosing a vein

Veins to avoid:
- Infection/inflammation evident
- Veins close to bruising and phlebitis
- Oedematous limbs (predisposed to complications as phlebitis and cellulitis)
- Areas of previous venepuncture (scar tissue)
- Thrombosed veins
- Do not use the affected arm in CVA or mastectomy patients
- A vein sited in the region of a drip site (may result in diluted samples)

Palpation to:
- Determine the location and condition of the veins
- Distinguishes veins from arteries and tendons
- Identifies the presence of valves

Healthy veins feel soft and bouncy and will refill when depressed

**VENEPUNCTURE: PRE-PROCEDURE CONSIDERATIONS**

Veins have layers:

Tunica intima (inner most – epithelial tissue)
Tunica media (muscle, nerve fibres)
Tunica adventitia (outer most – connective tissue)

Endothelium (Tunica Intima)
Internal Elastic Tissue
Smooth Muscle (Tunica Media)
External Elastic Tissue
Fibrous Connective Tissue (Tunica Adventitia)
Lumen
Flow
Vein

Figure 2: Vein structure.
http://www.med-ed.virginia.edu/courses/cell/handouts/images/BloodVessel_1.gif

**Veins**
Throughout out body but generally on arms
- Superficial veins
- Deep veins
Superficial most commonly selected – may use foot vein if necessary

Main veins of choice are:
- Median cubital vein
- Cephalic vein
- Basilic vein
- Metacarpal veins.
General choice: Median cubital vein (in antecubital fossa) as it is well supported by subcutaneous tissue.

**Veins in the Forearm**
Median cubital
Cephalic
Radial
Median antebrachial
Basilic
Ulnar

Figure 1 Veins. OpenStax College/CC BY
(https://creativecommons.org/licenses/by/3.0)

**Improving venous access**

1. Application of a Tourniquet
- Promotes venous distension
- Tight enough to impede venous return not arterial flow
- Placed 7–8 cm above venepuncture site
- Not be left on for longer than 1 minute (haemo-concentration/ pooling of the blood)

2. Opening and closing of the fist
- Muscles force blood into the veins and distension

3. Light tapping of the vein
- Can be painful in patients with fragile veins

4. The use of heat
- Warm pack (venodilatation and venous filling)

5. Lowering the arm below the level of the heart

**FIGURE 6.2** Venepuncture pre-procedure considerations

# VENEPUNCTURE: PROCEDURE

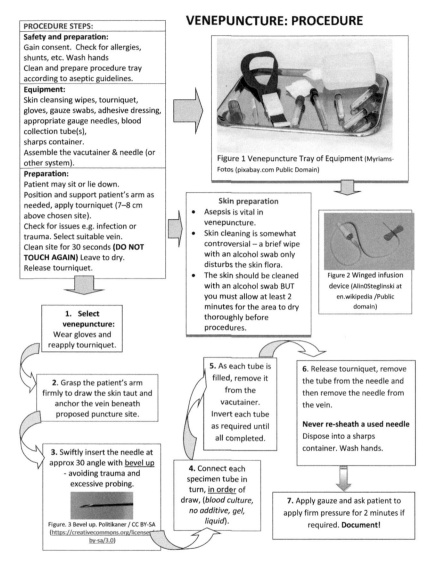

**PROCEDURE STEPS:**

**Safety and preparation:**
Gain consent. Check for allergies, shunts, etc. Wash hands
Clean and prepare procedure tray according to aseptic guidelines.

**Equipment:**
Skin cleansing wipes, tourniquet, gloves, gauze swabs, adhesive dressing, appropriate gauge needles, blood collection tube(s), sharps container.
Assemble the vacutainer & needle (or other system).

**Preparation:**
Patient may sit or lie down.
Position and support patient's arm as needed, apply tourniquet (7–8 cm above chosen site).
Check for issues e.g. infection or trauma. Select suitable vein.
Clean site for 30 seconds **(DO NOT TOUCH AGAIN)** Leave to dry.
Release tourniquet.

Figure 1 Venepuncture Tray of Equipment (Myriams-Fotos (pixabay.com Public Domain)

**Skin preparation**
- Asepsis is vital in venepuncture.
- Skin cleaning is somewhat controversial – a brief wipe with an alcohol swab only disturbs the skin flora.
- The skin should be cleaned with an alcohol swab BUT you must allow at least 2 minutes for the area to dry thoroughly before procedures.

Figure 2 Winged infusion device (Alin0Steglinski at en.wikipedia /Public domain)

1. **Select venepuncture:** Wear gloves and reapply tourniquet.

2. Grasp the patient's arm firmly to draw the skin taut and anchor the vein beneath proposed puncture site.

3. Swiftly insert the needle at approx 30 angle with <u>bevel up</u> - avoiding trauma and excessive probing.

Figure. 3 Bevel up. Politikaner / CC BY-SA (https://creativecommons.org/licenses/by-sa/3.0)

4. Connect each specimen tube in turn, <u>in order</u> of draw, (*blood culture, no additive, gel, liquid*).

5. As each tube is filled, remove it from the vacutainer. Invert each tube as required until all completed.

6. Release tourniquet, remove the tube from the needle and then remove the needle from the vein.

**Never re-sheath a used needle** Dispose into a sharps container. Wash hands.

7. Apply gauze and ask patient to apply firm pressure for 2 minutes if required. **Document!**

**FIGURE 6.3** Venepuncture procedure

# CANNULATION: PROCEDURE

### Why cannulate?
It is INVASIVE so good rationale is needed. For example:
- Fluid and electrolyte replacement
- Administration of medicines
- Administration of blood/blood products
- Administration of Total Parenteral Nutrition
- Haemodynamic monitoring

### Advantages:
- Immediate effect
- Control over the rate of administration
- Patient cannot tolerate drugs/fluids orally
- Some drugs cannot be absorbed by any other route

### Skin preparation
- Asepsis is vital in venepuncture.
- Skin cleaning – follow venepuncture notes.
- MUST allow 2 minutes for the area to dry thoroughly before procedures.

### What equipment do you need?
- Dressing tray (aseptic technique)
- Non sterile gloves/apron
- Cleaning wipes
- Gauze swab
- Appropriate IV cannula
- Tourniquet
- Dressing to secure cannula
- Alcohol wipes
- Saline flush and sterile syringe or fluid to be administered
- Sharps bins

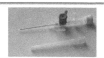

### Physical Preparation:
- Explain procedure with rationale and gain consent.
- Position the patient appropriately (non-dominant hand/arm).
- Support arm.
- Check for any contra-indications e.g. infection, damaged tissue, arterio-venous fistula etc.

### 1. Getting ready
Hand hygiene/prepare aseptic approach.
Remove the cannula from the packaging and check all parts are operational.
Loosen the white cap and gently replace it.

### 5. Completing procedure
Apply gentle pressure over the vein (beyond the cannula tip) remove the white cap from the needle.
Remove the needle from the cannula and dispose of it into a sharps container.
Attach the white lock cap.
Secure the cannula with an appropriate dressing.
Flush the cannula with 2–5 mls 0.9% Sodium Chloride or attach an IV giving set and fluid.

### 2. Site
Apply tourniquet and identify vein, clean the site as before.
Remove tourniquet and put on non-sterile gloves. Re-apply the tourniquet, 7–10 cm above site.

### 4. Advancing
Lower the cannula slightly ensure it enters the lumen.
Do not puncture exterior wall of the vessel.
Gently advance the cannula over the needle whilst withdrawing the guide, noting secondary flashback along the cannula.
Release the tourniquet.

### 3. Insertion
Remove the protective sleeve from the needle – do not touch it. With cannula in dominant hand, stretch the skin over the vein to anchor vein (do not re palpate the vein). Insert the needle (bevel up) at an angle of 10–30 degrees to the skin. Observe for blood in the flashback chamber.

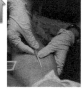

### 6. Governance
Document the procedure including:
Date & time, site and size of cannula, any problems encountered.
Review date (no longer than 72 hours).

**FIGURE 6.4** Cannulation procedure

# VESSEL HEALTH AND PRESERVATION: DECISION-MAKING

**Why a Framework?**
The UK Infection Prevention Society (IPS) produced a vessel health and preservation (VHP) framework (Hallam et al., 2016) following on from work by Moreau et al. (2015) addressing a range of issues:
- Junior staff
- Poor skill/technique
- Multiple attempts

**Decision Making Tool:** *similar to APIE (Assess, Plan, Implement, Evaluate)*
*Key areas:*
1. Is therapy required?
2. Correct line decision (peripheral versus central)
3. Vessel assessment
   a. Suitability for drugs and route
4. Re-evaluation of VAD

Vascular access devices (VADs) can be life-saving for patients or cause problems both minor or major:
- Phlebitis
- Thrombus
- Infection
- Damage to the vessel
- Blood stream infections (sepsis) (Moureau et al., 2012).

Implications for patients of failed cannulation or repeated siting of cannulae include:
- Pain
- Delayed IV fluids, antibiotics and analgesia
- Increased length of hospital stay
- Poor patient experience

**Individual Patient Choices:**
Patient preference/lifestyle (if longer term)
- Physical abnormalities/debilities
- Treatment specific routes (longer terms drugs)
- Past medical history (other access routes eg. Fistula

**Re-evaluation of VAD:**
Consider to continue with VAD or not:
**NO** = removal is recommended.
**YES** = then assessment considering:

- Presence or suspected infection
- Occlusion/thrombus at site
- Leakage
- Dislodgement
- Non-functioning and missing medications

| Peripheral vein assessment | | | | (based on Hallam, 2016) |
|---|---|---|---|---|
| | **1**<br>**Excellent** | **2**<br>**Good** | **3**<br>**Fair** | **4**<br>**Poor** | **5**<br>**None identifiable** |
| **Vein quality** | *4-5 palpable veins suitable* | *2-3 palpable veins suitable* | *1-2 palpable veins – may be small or scarred* | *Veins not palpable or needs infrared viewer* | *No visible veins* |
| **Duration** | Less 6 months (intermittent) | Less 4 months (intermittent) | 4 to 6 weeks (intermittent) | One off cannulation | Not suitable for cannulation |

**Cannula inserted by trained/authorised healthcare practitioners**

**FIGURE 6.5** Vessel health and decision-making

## COMPLICATIONS OF CANNULATION

**Inflammatory complications**
- **Insertion site infection:** colonisation by bacteria may be difficult to identify but relatively common.
- **Cellulitis:** inflammation of site not due to infection.
- **Air embolism** occurs when air enters the infusion line, although this is very rare – all lines are primed prior to use.
- **Haematoma** occurs when blood leaks out of the infusion site if on insertion the cannula has penetrated through the other side of the vessel wall.
- **Phlebitis** is common in IV therapy and can be caused in many ways. It is inflammation of a vein (redness and pain at the infusion site) – prevention can be using aseptic insertion techniques, choosing the smallest gauge cannula possible for the prescribed treatment, securing the cannula properly to prevent movement and carry out regular checks of the infusion site.

**Principles of care of a VAD**
- Prevent infection
- Maintain a closed IV system with few connections to reduce risk of contamination
- Maintain a patent device
- Prevent damage to device and equipment (Lister, Hofland and Grafton 2020)

**Integrity complications**
- **Infiltration** or 'tissuing' if infusion (fluid) leaks into the surrounding tissue. Could led to tissue necrosis.
- **Thrombolism/ thrombophlebitis:** small clot becomes detached from the sheath of the cannula or the vessel wall. Prevention is via flushing cannula regularly and consider re-siting the cannula if prolonged use is anticipated.
- **Extravasation** is the accidental administration of IV drugs into the surrounding tissue if the needle has punctured the vein. If with high osmolarity or chemotherapy drugs could be significant tissue destruction, and complications.
- **Bruising** commonly results from failed IV placement - particularly in the elderly and those on anticoagulant therapy.

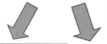

**Phlebitis Grading or Scoring Scale**
Two possible assessment scales include:

**Visual Infusion Phlebitis (VIP) scale** (Jackson, 1998):
**0** – site is healthy (no action)
**1** – one item (red or swelling) present (be alert and monitor)
**2** – two items of pain, erythema or swelling (resit e cannula)
**3** – three key signs or pain, erythema, and induration (resite cannula, moderate phlebitis)
**4** – extensive pain, erythema, induration (advanced, possibly treat but need to resite cannula)
**5** – all of above with pyrexia (treatment)
indicating presence of nothing to pain, redness, swelling, erythema and pyrexia.

**Infusion Nurses Scale (2011)** Grade 0 – No symptoms.
Grade 1 – Erythema at access site with or without pain.
Grade 2 – Pain at access site with erythema and/or oedema.
Grade 3 – Pain at access site with erythema and/or oedema, streak formation, palpable venous cord.
Grade 4 – Pain at access site with erythema and/or oedema, streak formation, palpable venous cord greater than 1 in in length; purulent drainage.

**Infection prevention in IV line management**
EPIC3 guidelines (Loveday et al, 2014) provide comprehensive recommendations for preventing healthcare acquired infections in hospital and other acute care settings based on the best currently available evidence.

- Replace all tubing when vascular device is changed.
- All IV giving sets for peripheral and central use should be changed every 72 hours unless more frequently is indicated clinically.
- Replace blood and blood products IV giving sets every 12 hours and after every second unit of blood.
- Discard intermittent infusions sets immediately after use.

**FIGURE 6.6** Complications of cannulation

**Activity: now test yourself**

1. Place these steps in the right order for obtaining a blood specimen by venepuncture:

   a) apply tourniquet

   b) puncture arm

   c) establish blood flow

   d) select a suitable vein

   e) remove needle

   f) release tourniquet

   g) fill and mix tubes.

2. When performing venepuncture the needle should always be inserted at the puncture site with the

   a) bevel side down

   b) bevel positioned away from the insertion site

   c) bevel side upward

   d) none of the above.

3. Thrombophlebitis is

   a) inflammation of a vein with formation of a clot

   b) inflammation of an artery with the formation of fibrin and collagen

    c)   inflammation of a capillary with the formation of a clot that moves

    d)   inflammation of a vein with formation of a bruise.

4.   Name three characteristics of a 'good vein'.

5.   Name three reasons why cannulation may be needed.

**Answers**

1. d) select a suitable vein; a) apply tourniquet; b) puncture arm; c) establish blood flow; g) fill and mix tubes; f) release tourniquet; e) remove needle.

2. c) bevel side upwards – also, insert the needle at approximately a 30-degree angle. Bevel orientation reduces trauma.

3. a) thrombophlebitis refers to two elements: clot and inflammation.

4. A good vein will be:

   • *large*

   • *easily accessible*

   • *relatively straight*

   • *away from any potentially harmful anatomy (such as a nerve or an artery)*

   • *palpable*

   • *firm and 'spongy'.*

5. Cannulation may be required for:

   • *fluid and electrolyte replacement*

   • *administration of medicines*

   • *administration of blood/blood products*

   • *administration of total parenteral nutrition*

   • *haemodynamic monitoring.*

## Reflection: ask yourself

1. What do I know now that I didn't know before?

2. What am I confused/unclear about?

3. What areas do I need to focus on?

4. My action plan for further learning (make objectives SMART – Specific/Measurable/Achievable/Realistic/Time-bound):

# Bibliography

Brekke, I. J., Puntervoll, L. H., Pedersen, P. B., Kellett, J., & Brabrand, M. (2019). The value of vital sign trends in predicting and monitoring clinical deterioration: a systematic review. *PloS One*, 14(1), e0210875. doi: 10.1371/journal.pone.0210875

Cardona-Morrell, M., Prgomet, M., Lake, R., Nicholson, M., Harrison, R., Long, J., Westbrook, J., Braithwaite, J., & Hillman, K. (2016). Vital signs monitoring and nurse-patient interaction: A qualitative observational study of hospital practice. *International Journal of Nursing Studies*, 56, 9–16. doi: 10.1016/j.ijnurstu.2015.12.007

Fleming et al. (2011). Normal ranges of heart rate and respiratory rate in children from birth to 18 years: a systematic review of observational studies. *Lancet* 377(9770), 1011–1018.

Global Initiative for Chronic Obstructive Lung Disease (GOLD) (2017). *Pocket Guide to COPD Diagnosis, Management, and Prevention. A Guide for Health Care Professionals.* Global Initiative for Chronic Obstructive Lung Disease, Inc. Available at https://goldcopd.org/wp-content/uploads/2016/12/wms-GOLD-2017-Pocket-Guide.pdf (Accessed 2nd August 2020).

Hallam, C., Weston, V., Denton, A., Hill, S., Bodenham, A., Dunn, H., Jackson, T. (2016). Development of the UK Vessel Health and Preservation (VHP) framework: a multi-organisational collaborative. *Journal of Infection Prevention* 17(2) 65–72. Available at https://doi.org/10.1177/1757177415624752 (Accessed 20th April 2020).

Jackson, A. (1998). Infection control: a battle in vein infusion phlebitis. *Nursing Times* 94: 4, 68–71.

Kim, W. Y., Lee, J., Lee, J., Jung, W. K., Kim, H. J., Huh, J. W., Lim, C., Koh, Y., & Hong, S. (2017). A risk scoring model based on vital signs and laboratory data predicting transfer to the intensive care unit of patients admitted to gastroenterology wards. *Journal of Critical Care*, 40, 213–217.

Lister, S., Hofland, J., Grafton, H. (2020). *The Royal Marsden Manual of Clinical Nursing Procedures (Royal Marsden Manual Series)* (10th edition). London: Wiley Blackwell and The Royal Marsden NHS Foundation Trust.

Mok, W., Wang, W., Cooper, S., Neo, E., Ang, K., & Ying Liaw, S. (2015). Attitudes towards vital signs monitoring in the detection of clinical deterioration: Scale development and survey of ward nurses. *International Journal of Quality in Health Care*, 27(3), 207–213.

Moureau, N. L., Trick, N., Nifong, T., Perry, C., Kelley, C., Leavett, M., Gordan, S. M., Wallace, J., Harvill, M., Biggar, C., Doll, M., Papke, L., Benton, L., Phelan, D. A. (2012). Vessel health and preservation (Part 1): a new evidence-based approach to vascular access selection and management. *Journal of Vascular Access* 13: 351–356. Available at https://doi.org/10.5301/jva.5000042 (Accessed 20th April, 2020).

National Institute for Health and Care Excellence (NICE) (2007). *Acutely Ill Patients in Hospital: Recognition of and Response to Acute Illness in Adults in Hospital*. London: NICE.

National Institute for Health and Care Excellence (NICE) (2011). *Hypertension: management of hypertension in adults in primary care*. CG no 127. London: NICE.

National Institute for Health and Care Excellence (NICE) (2013). *Fever in under 5s: assessment and management*. CG no 160. London: NICE.

National Institute for Health and Care Excellence (NICE) (2020). *Acutely Ill Adult in Hospital Overview*. London. Available at file:///C:/Users/tin a2/AppData/Local/Temp/acutely-ill-patients-in-hospital-acutely-ill-patients-in-hospital-overview-1.pdf (Accessed 22nd June, 2020).

National Patient Safety Agency (2007). *Safety First: one year on*. London: NPSA.

Nursing and Midwifery Council (NMC) (2018). *Future Nurse Proficiencies*. London. Available at https://www.nmc.org.uk/globalassets/sitedocuments/education-standards/future-nurse-proficiencies.pdf (Accessed 3rd July, 2020).

Pediatric advanced life support (PALS). *2015 Circulation*. Available at https://www.ahajournals.org/doi/10.1161/CIR.0000000000000266 (Accessed 14th August 2020).

Royal College of Nursing (2016a). *Rapid evidence review for the RCN infusion therapy standards: a summary*. London: The Royal College of Nursing.

Royal College of Nursing (2016b). *Competences: an education and training competence framework for peripheral venous cannulation in children and young people*. London: The Royal College of Nursing.

Royal College of Nursing (2017). *Standards for assessing, measuring and monitoring vital signs in infants, children and young people*. Available at https://www.rcn.org.uk/professional-development/publications/pub-005942 (Accessed 14th August, 2020).

Royal College of Physicians (2017). *National Early Warning Score (NEWS2): standardising the assessment of acute-severe illness in the NHS*. Report of a working party. London: Royal College of Physicians.

The Royal College of Medicine (2019). *Vital Signs in Adults: National Quality Improvement Project*. National Report 2018/2019.

# Index

Page numbers in *italics* denote figures.

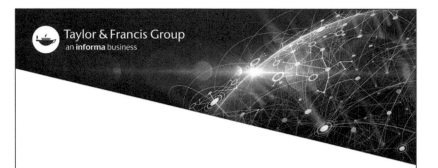